I0841287

The Monster's Weakness

How I overcame chronic migraine in one week by battling insulin resistance

BY PEARL HOWIE

Copyright © Pearl Howie 2023

All rights reserved

First Edition

The moral right of the author has been asserted

The right of Pearl Howie to be identified as the author of this book has been asserted by her in accordance with the Copyright, Design & Patents Act, 1988.

ISBN: 9798866756025

All rights reserved. Apart from any use permitted under UK copyright law, no part of this publication may be reproduced, stored or transmitted in any form or by any means without the prior permission in writing of the publisher or in the case of reprographic production in accordance with the terms of licences issued by the Copyright Licensing Agency.

Published by Pearl Escapes

www.pearlescapes.co.uk

pearl@pearlescapes.co.uk

Distributed in the UK by

Flying Machine Films Ltd.

Freedom Works, Metro House, Northgate,

Chichester PO19 1BJ, United Kingdom

Contents

Dedication

My optician.

Alex, if you hadn't waved the red flag,

would I ever have found the weakness?

Preface

I came to write this book because I was writing a different book (that will be coming out shortly). I started writing about health, because I was suffering from a period of the worst physical health I have ever experienced. But I wanted to talk about health from the point of view of a shaman or a wise woman, I wanted to talk about health as being mind, body and spirit, connected and interconnected, really just one thing after all.

I wanted to explain that, when we take care of our whole health - mind, body and spirit - that when we experience a challenge, whether it's an illness, a bereavement or a situation like Covid, we can survive it better. Instead of just focusing on what we could label physical health or mental health, what if we took care of ourselves, loved ourselves unconditionally?

Sadly, this week, Matthew Perry, star of "Friends", passed away and he reminds me so powerfully of other people who I've loved who I lost far, far too young. People who, whether or not they looked cool and fun and successful, were hurting dreadfully inside (and were often capable of dreadfully hurting people around them). Watching his old interviews, he talks about getting everything – the fame, the friends, the success he craved and realising that it didn't fill him up. Like that, we can often see people who seem to have it all – the millionaires, the politicians, the artists – people who seem to be role models and yet, they are far from healthy, far from happy.

I was living almost an opposite existence. My migraines were chronic and my quality of life was low, my physical health a daily battle. My income was also low, like a lot of people during a cost of living crisis, following a pandemic. I was just getting by, but I'm also a shaman. I've walked the walk, done the apprenticeship and so, my spiritual health was wonderful, my mental health, aside from the times that migraine and money knocked me over, was also good, my relationship with friends and family challenged by my constant migraines, but in some ways, stronger, at least with those friends and family members I managed to keep communicating with.

Recently, a friend of mine who is severely disabled wrote on LinkedIn about what was most important to keep him going. He said that it might surprise people to know that the most important thing was having strong and positive mental health.

One of my teachers, Don Miguel Ruiz, who has battled heart failure and is now the grateful recipient of a second heart transplant, talks often about the importance of will. Getting up and keeping going when the doctors have counted you out. I often thought about it, but I didn't know how to use my will, except in keeping going with the structured existence I had created to manage my migraines, taking various supplements, eating enough magnesium, trying to get enough sleep, drinking plenty of water and having supplies in for those long bouts. Was I supposed to use my will to nag the doctors for medication? Was I supposed to use my will to keep trying to work, booking appointments and interviews, even if I had to cancel so many times due to migraine? Was I supposed to use my will to just keep going… perhaps for another seven years of perimenopause and menopause?

So when I had (what I thought was) a different health emergency, when I thought I was pre-diabetic, it was in some ways an easy path, despite being physically hard and painful. I finally knew which way to go. Like doing the Camino de Santiago, the hardest part was getting to the beginning.

If you want to start right this second, you can always go straight to the plan – step by step chapter to plan your journey. But no matter where this journey takes you, you have to start from where you are.

Introduction

Migraine. It's a problem.

When you start asking the right questions, better questions, you start to realise what a big problem. I wish I could say that this solution, the way I battled migraine would work for everyone. I don't know that. But from piecing together the scientific studies and my own practical experience, what I can say is that this will probably work for a large number of migraine sufferers.

If you've ever had a migraine triggered by low blood sugar, improving your insulin sensitivity could prevent you suffering again. (And you, like me, may not be aware of all the times a migraine may have been triggered by either low or high blood sugar – even, at times, independently of what you've eaten.)

What I can also say is that it will help almost everyone's general health and that's a huge positive (especially compared to many of the other migraine treatments out there that come with serious side effects and negative impact on the rest of our health).

This is the way I found to battle *my* monster. My chronic migraines.

In all good "creature features" the town, the city, the world is on the run from a vile creature… body snatchers, nasty scuttly things, Triffids… and then someone discovers the monster's weakness. At last, there's hope. Whether it's a certain frequency of sound that renders them immobile or, like "The Wizard of Oz", a bucket of water chucked over the head of The Wicked Witch of the West, that discovery, often an accidental discovery, gives the people back their freedom.

Migraine is a monster, it destroys lives. I don't think we have numbers for suicide but I'm in no doubt that each year, people take their own lives rather than keep suffering. I've thought about it. Even promised myself in the worst times that I'd put myself out of my misery when I was able to, when the migraine was over. Instead, of course, the sun came up and I found my joy again. For me it was a lie, but for others, perhaps not.

There are guesstimates like, migraines cost the UK economy £2 billion a year. Or, from the Global Burden of Disease study of 2019 ("the largest and most comprehensive effort to quantify health loss across places and over time" including "more than 3.5 billion estimates of … 369 diseases and injuries … in 204 countries and territories") that migraine is the second cause of disability in the world and the first among young females. (From "Migraine remains second among the world's causes of disability, and first among young women: findings from GBD2019" T. J. Steiner, L. J. Stovner, R. Jensen, D. Uluduz & Z. Katsarava on behalf of Lifting The Burden: the Global Campaign against Headache published 2 December 2020 in The Journal of Headache and Pain.)

Roughly 80% of patients seen for migraine in Neurology in the UK are women going through perimenopause and menopause – because that's when it really bites (especially in my case).

It affects 1 in 3 women and 1 in 7 men. Professor Peter

Goadsby (winner of the Brain Prize for his work on CGRP, calcitonin gene related peptides and ways to inhibit them to prevent migraine) puts it so well in his comments on migraine, that although we are working in the UK, migraine also affects millions, or maybe even billions in the developing world, who are also having to deal with the hardest ways of life, such as fetching water and firewood.

I lived with my monster for 40 years. I didn't even give it a name for the first 10 years. They were just headaches. It was only when they started making me vomit, I realised they might be migraines. And they were not that frequent and not that problematic. Mine were often a Friday night occurrence, when I'd had a busy week, or once a month for about 8 hours. They were a pain, but they didn't stop me living my life. I often had migraines after long flights, when I didn't eat properly, when it was hot and I got dehydrated. All the common causes. For almost 40 years, I never saw a doctor, was never part of the statistics. Like most, I discovered Migraleve, thought it was brilliant, took it for a bit, then realised it wasn't that great because of the codeine, became drug free and just naturally found my way to tiptoe around the monster when it was likely to be troublesome.

Then, through a combination of Covid, lockdown, perimenopause, lockdown, Covid vaccinations, lockdown, stress, lockdown, hot flushes… my monster turned into chronic migraine. Everywhere, all day, the low pain days where it was only a 1 or 2 not even registered on my migraine chart. The days that meant I could not deny it was chronic, where the pain was a 3, 4 or even an 8 (thankfully it hasn't reached a 9 or 10 in years), the days when I couldn't get out of bed, or eat…

It's hard to talk about. It's not just the pain, or the nausea, what still makes me sad are the 50th birthday parties I had to call and say I couldn't attend at the last minute. The friends I hurt. The way I shut my life down, not planning, because inevitably, even if it was a Zoom interview, I'd have to cancel because of migraine. My business – my trainings… I gave up organising. It was too much work to have to cancel at the last minute. The last thing that remained was caring for my family when I could, and teaching one Zumba Gold class over Zoom a week – when I could. The only silver lining was that I managed to move house in the middle of it, because of a brief reprieve from migraine and found myself living by the sea, where I could walk and try to get a bit healthy, where, when it was very hot, I could go swimming in the evening, which really helped with lurking migraine. I found a little bit of heaven to get me through hell.

Chronic migraine often meant not being able to look at emails for three days or more, not great when you are looking for work. I always padded my deadlines with a few days for safety, but when the migraines would last six days, it's a miracle that I didn't let more people down.

Chronic migraine meant having to think about the paperwork required to become officially classified as disabled, in order to get support. I knew I was living on the edge, it was like I was holding my breath as my monthly cycles got closer together in perimenopause, so that my 6 day migraines were only 10 days apart, fearing that soon there would be no time for me to come up for air.

Migraine, my monster, was closing in.

The Optician Waves the Red Flag

The link to blood sugar was only flagged by my optician when I went for a check up, only a year after my contact lens check up. My eyesight had shifted so much that she wanted my doctor to check my blood sugar, as blood sugar spikes can cause eyesight to suddenly deteriorate (although it can recover when the blood sugar is controlled).

At this point, I had changed my GP in order to try to get more help with my migraines.

I was on high dose B2 and eating magnesium rich foods, as well as on Menopace and drinking buckets of green tea (having quit all tea and coffee – even decaff to help with the migraines).

We'd had one appointment and he had suggested three possible medications – topiramate (a reasonably effective preventative but with an estimated 30% risk of causing depression), propranolol (another preventative, with risk of weight gain, also not to be used for those who have ever had serious depression or considered self harm) and metoclopramide to be used for nausea (with some rarer side effects, but only to be taken occasionally).

He wasn't too worried about the fact I was already clinically obese, possibly the heaviest I've ever been. Neither was I. I had put on a lot of weight before, notably after I gave a kidney to my brother and had to rehab my body, and I knew I could lose the weight through Zumba, as I'd done before, if only I could stop having migraines enough to do it.

As the optician requested, a HbA1c, the standard for testing for diabetes and blood sugar issues was booked… but then I ended up in A&E with a migraine and vomiting so violent that I was also bleeding (apparently it's common and the doctor wasn't worried, but I was!) I was also terrified that I might be having a stroke as I found it so hard to move and speak. He ordered a blood sugar test as well, and a kidney function test, as I just have one kidney. By the time I left, he was pleased to report that all my tests were fine, although my blood sugar was just over the normal limit. I was also relaxed after he gave me a stroke check.

In that moment, despite being incapacitated by migraine, by my monster once again, I knew one thing. I had to get moving. I knew, from all my training with Zumba, that exercise improves insulin sensitivity. And I knew that even if my migraines were awful, they weren't going to kill me, but allowing myself to become clinically obese through inactivity and eating junk food (because oven chips were often the only thing I could face) really could. I did not want to be diabetic.

This is like the moment in the movie, when the people have been hiding from the monster, slowly running out of food and water, and then someone gets hurt and they realise they have to risk going into town to get medicine. (And that's how they discover the monster's weakness.)

Let's Go!

I never thought that I would become a fitness instructor. I had a painful history with PE at school. I was the loser, the last, the one who didn't even get the bronze certificate in Athletics. I was less a runner and jumper and more a sit in the library-er. But I always loved to dance. And although I was socially awkward at that age, when I went to parties, I was the first one on the dancefloor.

After I donated a kidney to my brother, my body was a mess. (I even wrote a book about that – my first non-fiction.) The physio came the day after the surgery and told me she was going to get me up, walking and sitting in the chair. I told her I was in too much pain. She nodded. I had an epidural and so many wires, tubes and a drip. Nothing would stop her. She had warned me in pre-op. 'We're going to make you wiggle your toes when you come out of surgery and the next day we're going to come and get you up. You won't want to, but you have to.'

Pain just really isn't a big enough word. But they have to do it. Because of circulation and risks of blood clots and just making your body move.

Then there's pain at night, and the referred pain, when your lower back makes it feel like your arm is about to fall off. Drugs aren't enough, and epidurals fail. And you feel all the pain of the scalpel the day before and you think you're going to die.

Then they give you too many tablets and you vomit and you think you're going to die.

Then they tell you they can't give you any more painkillers. (After you've agreed they can take out the sodding, ineffectual epidural.) And it's two days on paracetamol before they give you a decent painkiller.

Getting fit after that experience was a long road. I often went two steps forward and three steps back. I was impatient to get on with my life. I would do a few too many sit ups in the gym and then have abdominal muscle spasms for days. It took a lot for me to learn to go easy. Recovery was measured in months (I wasn't allowed to drive for the first month) and, when I went back to work as a temp, I only managed a few days before they let me go - I had to take so many painkillers to sit in a chair all day that I did not do my best work!

But what really upset me was that when I tried to dance in a club, my right hip (where I'd had the surgery) would not move when I wanted it to. I'd always been a great dancer, even if I was rubbish at everything else. I couldn't bear having that taken away from me.

So I went to belly dancing at my gym – and even though it took weeks and hours of drills, of body rolls and hip lifts and even a bit of veil dancing… I got it back. I got my body back.

Sadly, a few years later, I put my back out – probably trying to move a washing machine. I spent around 12 weeks hardly able to get out of bed, but the doctor could only offer painkillers.

In desperation I went to my gym again, to see a sports physio.

She gave me some exercises to do three times a day, to strengthen my core muscles. As much as it hurt, I could feel my back healing a little bit more every time, within days I was on the mend.

I still do those exercises – every morning (well, when my monster allows) – to protect my back and keep me moving (I even throw in some Kundalini yoga moves).

I kept going to the gym, I had managed to get to a really healthy weight, but then I seemed to plateau, and even though I was going to the gym every morning, I was putting on a huge amount of weight and so I tried Zumba. Six months later, I quit my job, because I realised how unhappy I was (migraines showed up too, to prove the point) and decided I would figure something else out, and part of it would be being a Zumba Instructor.

When I was about to do my Zumba Instructor training, disaster struck, and I threw my back out again. Luckily, I was still working and covered by private healthcare, so I took myself to a sports physio again. I was terrified of being told not to do Zumba, it was such a big part of my life (a chiropractor had even told me before that Zumba was really bad for my hips and I shouldn't be doing it at my age – so not true, it's one of the best things you can do to avoid having to have a hip replacement). My sports physio was fantastic and told me that I could do whatever I wanted, provided I kept my core muscles strong. He gave me a bit of massage (that was so painful it made me want to throw up) and then made me do the worst exercises he could throw at me to strengthen those muscles.

I really hated him. He worked me to the point of collapse so many times, I was in such pain, but I knew I needed it, knew that it was a temporary thing, and essential if I wanted to get on with my life.

Over time, as a Zumba Instructor, I worked with almost everyone, children with severe disabilities, dementia patients, people suffering from MS. I was so privileged to be invited into their world, to deliver whatever I could with music and movement to help them feel better, to have a laugh and most importantly, to party. But I think I was good at it because I knew what it was like, to be the person in the chair, to be in such terrible pain, to not be able to move, to walk. I was lucky to have been able to rehab my body, so lucky, and I wanted to do whatever I could to help them, knowing that miracles are possible.

I think Zumba saved my life. Losing weight, reminding myself what it felt like to be happy, reawakening my soul, allowing me to leave… work at first and then, six years after training as an instructor, home, London and travel the world and embrace my destiny.

Three years after that departure, I was arriving home, close to most of my family just before Covid hit (I think I actually had Covid in my body when I moved in) to what should have been a winter let, but which became my home for three years. I had already started doing my Zumba Instructor videos online to get myself fit.

When Covid really hit in 2020, Zumba Home Office gave us special permission to teach online and I set up my Monday morning Zumba Gold class on Zoom. I woke up on the Sunday morning, the day before I started, with Covid symptoms for the second time, and then the government announced the first lockdown.

Teaching Zumba classes, I discovered, was the key to recovering from Covid – keeping going when all I wanted to do was lie down and sleep. (It also helped that my bathroom was downstairs and bedroom upstairs, perhaps those stairs saved my life by keeping me using my lungs.)

January 2021 was in some ways the worst for me. I hadn't realised that I was starting perimenopause, but I was soaking up the news and enduring lockdown and, for the first time in my life, I was scared of the police. Bear in mind that I was living in a tiny village, where we all said hello to each other, but the new rules of Covid, which I'd misstepped by accident at least once or twice, made me feel that just leaving the house, or sitting on a bench (which we were forbidden to do by law) when my energy levels gave out, as they seemed to do without warning, could have me in trouble with the police. It seems, in one light, crazy, in another… it was only a short time after that when a young girl was abducted and murdered by a policeman. We were living under martial law and as we all know: "Power corrupts, absolute power corrupts absolutely."

I could have done Zumba for myself at home, inside. I wish I had. But I was just hanging on, holding my breath, waiting for things to get better.

Friends and colleagues were starting new live classes, then getting them shut down again in the months before and the months after. All I could do was watch, wait and wake up on Monday and force myself to cheer up my Zumba gang, and thank goodness, cheer myself up in the process.

At a certain point, I realised that doing an hour of exercise each day was the key to not feeling so awful. Fatigue, migraine, nausea, dizziness – it was impossible to tell whether it was caused by long Covid, Covid vaccinations, stress, perimenopause, menstruation or migraine. But an hour walking around the village, when I was able, definitely helped. If I couldn't do an hour, I'd do twenty minutes, or fifteen, sometimes twice a day, I'd set a timer on my phone and head off.

When I moved house, three years later, I didn't need a timer for my walks, walking to and from the beach was about an hour round trip and I always wanted to go. My health improved slowly, my migraines were not so bad… until the summer.

When I panicked about my blood sugar, I decided I would try to do two Zumba sessions per week. I was already doing one on Monday (when I could) and so, if I could do one on Wednesday or Thursday, even if I couldn't manage to do anything for the rest of the day (Zumba often triggered or put me on the edge of a migraine on a Monday) it would help my insulin sensitivity. Then perhaps I could gradually build up to three or four as my body got used to it again? If it didn't make my migraines too much worse…

I managed two in the first week, that week of my optician's appointment… and then ended up in A&E two days later with a menstrual migraine. In total, that migraine took me out of the game for six days, although I did manage to make it to the beach on the last day.

I decided that if I wanted to tackle my blood sugar problems, the only way to do it was to adopt the adage of a Scottish clan: "If I can, I will." I would treat Zumba like physio, like my back exercises in the morning. I would make it my first priority and have faith that I would improve my health enough for it not to be the only thing I could do in a day.

I did three days of Zumba back to back, Thursday, Friday, Saturday and then gave myself a rest day on the Sunday. My body hurt, my muscles ached, I was constantly on the verge of a full blow migraine, headachey and even so nauseous at one point I had to take one of my anti-nausea tablets (metoclopramide). But I did it. I figured I was also suffering from detox headaches, so upped the green tea and tried to eat more healthily – more vegetables, nuts and beans, all low GI foods to try to make me more insulin sensitive.

Monday, I taught my class, then Tuesday a bad migraine struck. I could tell by the symptoms that it was another menstrual migraine (even though I didn't have a period this time) the nausea was terrible. I used the anti-nausea tablets and finally managed to sleep. I woke up at 1pm (12 hours after it started) and I was okay. I had a 12 hour migraine instead of a six day one. This was progress. I even managed a walk to the beach in the afternoon.

The next day, I did Zumba… and the next, and the next… each day I woke up feeling better, more myself.

From the Thursday morning when I decided to do Zumba every day I could, to the next Wednesday, I had one 12 hour migraine (and many, many low grade migraines triggered by exercise) and since then, the monster has quietened.

At first, I joked to myself, "Well I haven't killed it, but I've scared it off with the Zumba music!"

But then I sat on the bus and rode all the way without feeling car sick.

I cooked healthy dinners and had leftovers in the fridge (previously, I'd stopped making or buying anything that couldn't be quickly frozen, because I was so often nauseous, I had to keep throwing food away). I started to think about making plans to see friends once again.

I keep reminding myself that it is early days, that I felt like this when I gave up coffee and improved for a while, or started B2 and improved for a while, or increased my magnesium and felt better for a while… but I feel in my bones this is different. I feel that this is the monster's weakness.

Placebos are hugely effective in migraine studies – often a success result of 40%, because migraine is so linked to stress and so, fear.

If this is a placebo, I say, I'll keep it.

But the scientist part of me wants to dig, wants to know why this is working, wants to know what's going on in my body, why my attempt to increase insulin sensitivity is having such a dramatic effect (within one week!) on my monster, my migraines. Not just for other people and to share this, but because I want to keep doing the right things – I want my life back! And I'm going to do everything I can to keep it!

What's the Deal With Insulin and Insulin Resistance?

Insulin is the substance produced by the body which moves sugar or rather glucose (which all carbohydrates are converted into when digested) from your bloodstream into your cells. It's what stops you from having so much sugar in your blood that you get sick (or die). It's what stops you from having so much sugar in your blood that your eyesight goes crazy – like mine did or you have symptoms like nausea, dizziness and even fatigue (I know, strange for a blood sugar spike, right?)

Insulin sensitivity is when our cells respond well to insulin, bringing glucose from the bloodstream into the cells where it is stored or used. Insulin resistance is the opposite – poor insulin sensitivity.

On the other side, insulin works with another hormone - glucagon, which triggers the liver to convert stored glucose into a usable form and release it into the bloodstream, keeping our blood sugar at a safe level, stopping it from getting too low and causing other health issues (like fainting!)

A healthy system is one in which our body maintains enough insulin sensitivity to prevent it having to struggle to produce enough insulin to keep our blood sugar level. It also means that we're less likely to feel unwell from low blood sugar, because the body is also better at releasing glucose back into the blood stream when it's needed.

This is critical for migraines and for maintaining a healthy weight because then we don't always have to "top up" by having a snack (healthy or otherwise) when our blood sugar starts to get low – our body will naturally and easily access stored glucose in order to keep our blood sugar at the right level.

When you don't produce insulin or not enough insulin to manage that sugar/glucose, you are diabetic.

Type 1 diabetes is when someone can't produce insulin and people are often born with that condition.

Type 2 diabetes has different causes and, for most people, it's caused by being on the same road as me – not enough exercise, stress, hormonal issues and eating poorly so that we put on weight, and struggle with high and low blood sugar, until eventually, we have so much insulin resistance that our body can't produce enough insulin and we have to supplement it by taking medication.

But it's not just eating that affects our blood sugar so much, drops in oestrogen, lack of sleep and stress can all send our blood sugar up – it's no wonder that insulin sensitivity tends to go down during perimenopause and menopause.

There are also a whole host of things that affect our blood sugar, making it go up or down (these are some examples from the US' Centers for Disease Prevention and Control):

High sugar levels can come from sunburn, dehydration, artificial sweeteners, coffee (even black coffee), skipping breakfast in the morning can cause higher blood sugars after lunch and dinner, time of day (it can be harder to control blood sugar later in the day – perhaps why we used to say, 'Eat like a king at breakfast, a prince at lunch and a pauper in the evening.') and shifts in hormones throughout the day and night.

Conversely low sugar levels can be caused by things like extreme heat.

As the pain of sunburn causes stress, which can cause high blood sugar, it leads me to wonder if pain is more of a factor in creating high blood sugar than we recognise – pain like migraines or other serious medical conditions? Could these be more important on the path to obesity and type 2 diabetes than we have appreciated?

For someone who is diabetic, a low blood sugar or "hypo" – hypoglycaemic episode can be very serious, it can cause a whole host of symptoms – "feeling shaky, feeling disorientated, sweating, being anxious or irritable, going pale, palpitations and a fast pulse, lips feeling tingly, blurred vision, being hungry, feeling tearful, tiredness, having a headache, lack of concentration or even night sweats." Sourced from diabetes.org.uk, the website of Diabetes UK.

For someone who has migraines, especially when they're worsening for whatever reason migraines get worse at times, we're often ready to have a coffee or a sugary snack to prevent the dip in blood sugar that can trigger a migraine, and that, in turn, puts pressure on our body to use more insulin to store the excess glucose we've consumed, making us more insulin resistant.

The more inefficient our system is at managing blood sugar, the more inefficient it can become, unless we start doing the work to get it back in balance. (Sadly, this is like a lot of systems and organs in the body, once things start to deteriorate, it puts more pressure on and causes more deterioration. For example, kidney problems, which often result from diabetes, can cause high blood pressure, which puts more pressure on the kidney… it's so important to try to tackle these problems early, because while we say prevention is better than cure, sometimes there is no cure.)

Fat cells are naturally less responsive to insulin, so having a lot of white fat cells (like me!) means that my body is less responsive to insulin. I'm around two stone over the borderline for clinical obesity, so I'm pretty sure that's a big factor for me, and also for the great proportion of people who are developing or have already developed type 2 diabetes.

When we go through periods of stress or illness, our insulin sensitivity can decrease, and this should correct itself when we get past that period, but it does lead me to wonder, what can a pandemic of several years, when you're living in perpetual stress, do to the body's insulin sensitivity?

Unsurprisingly, eating a lot of sugar (actual sugar) and carbohydrates with a high glycaemic index (GI) (I'll explain more about that when we talk about healthy eating) puts a lot more pressure on our body to use insulin, because we're dumping a lot into our bloodstream in a short time. Whereas, when we eat low GI foods, like most fruit and vegetables and even fats and protein, we slow down the digestive process, give our body a break and we're less likely to make our body insulin resistant.

We believed that insulin was only produced in the islets of Langerhans in the pancreas – some things you don't forget from Biology "A" Level – but "recent evidence has shown that low concentrations are also found in certain neurons of the central nervous system" ("Role of Insulin in Health and Disease: An Update" by Md Saidur Rahman et al, 2021) which, again, makes me question the relationship of insulin sensitivity and migraine, as it is a neurological condition.

Even the experts still don't know all of the things that insulin does, like a lot of hormones. We understand what we think is the most important or life-threatening aspect of insulin resistance, but we've still got a long way to go to understand it all. We have to work with what we've got (and perhaps do a few of our own experiments!)

The Science

According to my GP, my HbA1c is perfect. Not good, not just not pre-diabetic, but about as good as it gets.

According to the duty doctor I consulted with last week, blood sugar spikes (or hyperglycaemia) are impossible if you have a good HbA1c.

A HbA1c is a way of measuring your average blood glucose (sugar) levels for the last two to three months.

From Lab Tests Online:

"Some of the glucose in your blood binds to haemoglobin (the protein that carries oxygen in your red blood cells). This combination of glucose and haemoglobin is called haemoglobin A1c (HbA1c). The amount of HbA1c formed is directly related to the average concentration of glucose in your bloodstream. Red blood cells live for 2–3 months, and because of this, the amount of HbA1c in your blood reflects the average level of glucose in your blood during the last 2-3 months. If your diabetes is not well controlled, your blood glucose levels will be high causing higher HbA1c levels."

It's important to remember (and I am a mathematician by training) that an average is just that, a number which reflects a levelling out of the highs and lows into one… average.

Or to put it another way, as my GP said, 'Yes of course you can have highs naturally. If there was a lion in this room your blood sugar would be through the roof because of your hormones.' And there's the answer to many of our blood sugar issues – not diet, but hormones.

When oestrogen drops, as it does at menstruation, ovulation and, of course, over time, during perimenopause, our drop in blood sugar causes… a spike in blood sugar. At exactly the same time as I experience my worst migraine symptoms.

You could ask, how it is possible to have had such spikes since puberty, those 40 years, without experiencing these kind of migraines? Well, because insulin sensitivity goes down during perimenopause. Even for someone who doesn't experience migraines, those sugar spikes can cause nausea, fatigue and dizziness. The same symptoms which are common during perimenopause and menopause.

Also, our insulin sensitivity goes down when we are inactive (whether due to migraine, weather or lockdown) when we eat a diet of food that has a high GI or glycaemic index, i.e. that our body absorbs the sugar (which actually includes starch) from very quickly – foods like sugar, white potatoes, white bread, even fruit juice. That low insulin sensitivity is also linked to being overweight, having more belly fat and more fat in general (but that could also be because of the inactivity and diet). (Which came first, the chicken or the egg? In this case I'm pretty sure it was that damn lockdown.)

Of course, it's not just female hormones that change blood sugar. Stress causes cortisol, which also raises blood sugar. (Stress like a global pandemic.)

Another classic cause of migraine.

Lack of sleep also causes blood sugar spikes, which, when the number one symptom of perimenopause and menopause is troubled sleep, makes us understand why we could be experiencing higher blood sugar, symptoms of hyperglycaemia (high blood sugar) and migraine at this time. Or indeed any time that we experience lack of sleep (like jet lag).

Another classic cause of migraine is low blood sugar – we know this and advice is often to eat snacks to keep the blood sugar level, but remember that our ability to handle low blood sugar is also affected when we build insulin resistance, so by battling insulin resistance we also decrease our tendency to have migraines because of low blood sugar.

To put this another way. When we suffer from migraines, especially chronic migraines, we are on edge, waiting for the monster to appear, so at the first inkling, the first rustle of the trees, we eat something to increase our blood sugar. This works to keep the monster at bay, but by increasing our blood sugar in the short term, we can also increase our insulin resistance in the long term, making the monster bigger. Does that make sense?

Building our insulin sensitivity, through exercise, healthy eating and also, by what comes naturally from doing that - maintaining a healthy weight and having less body fat, helps us to manage both natural high and low blood sugars – it allows our body to get our blood sugar back to a manageable level without struggling to produce more and more insulin, and critically for migraine sufferers, without triggering migraines.

One of the great things is that so much research has been done on migraines in the last few years, and when you start asking the right questions, you find the answers. So, I found this:

The study by Mona Ali et al on "The potential impact of insulin resistance and metabolic syndrome on migraine headache characteristics" published by BMC Neurology, 12 November 2022. (You can read it in its entirety online.)

Two small groups of people – one suffering from migraine and the other not – were studied using the following tests and measurements: waist circumference, fasting blood glucose, fasting insulin, high-density lipoprotein cholesterol level, and triglycerides, and HOMA-IR.

Unlike the HbA1c, the HOMA-IR (Homeostatic Model Assessment for Insulin Resistance) is a much more sophisticated test. According to Health Matters:

"When insulin resistance is identified early, it can be reversed. Using the HOMA-IR to identify subtle insulin resistance, even before it is evident in more traditional screening measures like hemoglobin HA1c (HA1c) and fasting blood sugar.

The HOMA-IR tool is a validated, non-invasive tool to assess the relationship between glucose and insulin. If elevated, it can guide you to make diet and lifestyle changes that will bring your HOMA-IR score down into the insulin-sensitive range, lose weight, and improve your health."

"What are some insulin resistance symptoms? The answer is there isn't any until it's too late, as you don't really feel insulin resistance. This is the same as hyperglycemia, where you don't really feel it until it damages your organs or is high enough to give you acidosis.

What is insulin resistance – is it a separate disease? Well, while we address it like an illness – there are drugs and interventions – it's more a state that precedes more severe metabolic disorders, such as diabetes. It's also usually paired with other cardiovascular risk factors, like obesity, lack of physical activity, high blood pressure, and hyperlipidemia. Early intervention and following the doctor's orders are key to saving yourself from serious consequences, such as blindness or kidney failure."

Getting back to the migraine study (although you might need to take a moment to digest those warnings about blindness and kidney failure – you can see why it had me running to call Renal to ask them to check my kidney function over the last few years – as a kidney donor, they check me out once a year) the overall conclusion was this:

"Insulin resistance and metabolic syndrome are more common in migraine patients than in healthy controls. The severity and impact of migraine attacks are higher in patients with insulin resistance than in those without."

If I had any doubts about the relationships between insulin sensitivity and migraine, what makes me even more positive (aside from the scientific studies) are the other common causes of migraine and the anomalies:

Alcohol is another cause of migraine. From Mount Sinai: "Drinking alcohol can cause low or high blood sugar."

Caffeine – for which there are as many studies showing it is beneficial to insulin sensitivity as there are saying it is harmful. In the same way, coffee has often been a favourite method of pain relief for migraineurs but, for me, on the days when I was nauseous, I couldn't keep down coffee and so suffered even worse from caffeine withdrawal. Giving it up certainly improved my migraines for a decent period of time.

But now let's get on to the fun stuff – how do we increase insulin sensitivity and battle insulin resistance, and how do we do it really, really quickly?!

More interesting studies

"Chronic migraine in women is associated with insulin resistance: a cross-sectional study" by A. Fava et al published in European Journal of Neurology, February 2014.

"Insulin Sensitivity is Impaired in Patients with Migraine" by I Rainero et al published by Sage Journals, August 2005.

How To Increase Insulin Sensitivity (SI)

(SI is how insulin sensitivity is abbreviated in research studies. Not confusing at all then.)

So how do we battle insulin resistance or increase insulin sensitivity and what have we been doing that has got us into this situation in the first place?

One of the first things to remember about common advice we get from our doctors and health services is that there is a focus on what can be easily seen and measured. There's an assumption that if someone's (my) HbA1c is okay, there isn't a blood sugar issue – but we've seen from other tests and research that that's not true.

Because there's also a link between obesity and blood sugar, often the first advice we get is to lose weight or even to reduce belly fat – those things are part of the overall picture, but they are very much the end result of increasing exercise and changing diet, and something we don't want to focus on too soon, because it's putting the cart before the horse!

Let's look at the NHS advice to avoid type 2 diabetes and reduce insulin resistance (according to the NHS, this single issue accounts for 10% of the NHS annual budget – and that's not even including people who are pre-diabetic, like me).

- Do around 150 minutes exercise per week

- Stop smoking

- Reduce or stop drinking alcohol

- Eat more healthily

- Lose weight

They are all pretty reasonable suggestions, but for me, not drinking or smoking and already doing, some days, at least 150 minutes of walking per *day*, and feeling so nauseous, this advice was just frustrating and not very inspiring.

When I started doing Zumba every day, it was in desperation, just knowing that it was a way I had lost a lot of weight before. But when it started working so quickly, I took another look at why – and looked around for more research.

From "Effect of Physical activity on Insulin Resistance, Inflammation and Oxidative Stress in Diabetes Mellitus" by Vighnesh Vetrivel Venkatasamy et al, 2013, published in the National Library of Medicine:

"A single bout of moderate intensity exercise can increase the glucose uptake by at least 40%." (Glucose uptake is another measure of how well our body is responding to insulin.)

"Glucose uptake remains elevated for up to 120 minutes after physical activity… Insulin sensitivity increases for at least 16 hours post-exercise. This is observed in healthy individuals as well as subjects with type 2 diabetes."

Apparently just one exercise session increases insulin sensitivity, helping us to maintain a healthy blood sugar where it might spike or dip due to stress, lack of sleep, hormone changes and what we eat. (You notice I put that last?) AND, when we do a training session, our bodies keep building insulin sensitivity for another 16 or more hours!

From "Update on the effects of physical activity on insulin sensitivity in humans" by Stephen R Bird1 and John A Hawley, 2016, published by BMJ Open Sport & Exercise Medicine.

"Some studies report exercise-induced benefits to SI that are independent of habitual diet and weight loss, while others indicate an association with fat reduction, hence the debate over the relative importance of PA (physical activity) and weight loss continues."

"A dose effect may be evident, with greater exercise volumes and higher exercise intensities, including high intensity interval training (HIIT) or sprint interval training (SIT), producing greater benefits to SI.

The combination of aerobic exercise training and REX (resistance exercise) may be more effective than either exercise mode alone."

So, what I was learning was, the intensity and also the "intervality", the mixed bag of exercise that Zumba is, was getting the best result for me. Not just in terms of intensity, because I was really struggling with the workout, but also the fact that it includes weight training – or rather body weight training – using the weight of my arms to workout, or indeed my entire body weight every time I tried to jump (or skip when jumping was too much).

And by exercising each day I was effectively giving my insulin sensitivity a 16 hour workout!

I also found online advice that recommended exercising strenuously at least five days a week, although I had set myself the target of every day, just because I could never tell when a migraine would knock me out for a day… or two… or six.

I also discovered that just three days of inactivity can reduce our insulin sensitivity. This wasn't a problem when my migraines would only last 8 hours, but as they got longer… some even as long as 7 days, I could see where my insulin sensitivity would have decreased just because I couldn't get out of bed.

But, as I started to figure things out, it gave me hope, not only that I was doing the right thing, but that, provided I could manage to exercise every third day, if I did get knocked out by a migraine, I wouldn't lose the insulin sensitivity I had gained.

It also made sense that the times my migraines had eased off in the summer were the days when it was so hot that I went out for a beach swim in the evening. Although swimming can be relaxing, I was so out of shape that each session (and the walk home) were as much as I could manage and, for me, pretty high intensity.

Having learned that fat cells have lower insulin sensitivity than other cells, for example, muscle, I also knew that building muscle, I was, cell by cell, making my body more insulin sensitive. Even without losing weight, my body was changing enough to become much, much healthier.

Healthy enough to improve the way I was eating… but I'll leave that to another chapter, first…

What Kind of Exercise and Why?

We have a saying in Zumba (especially Zumba Gold which is the program where we can adapt the workout for people with different abilities) that "all movement is good". It's worth remembering that what is the right exercise for one person is too much or not enough for someone else.

Looking back at the scientific studies in the last chapter, we saw that HIIT - high intensity interval training (or Sprint Training) seemed to be the most effective kind of exercise to improve insulin sensitivity, but let's put a pin in that for a moment and take a broader look at exercise before we look closer at HIIT and similar types of exercise and why they might be the most beneficial.

If you go online, you'll find that almost every kind of exercise is good for increasing insulin sensitivity. I think the trick is to do enough for you personally.

There was a time when a walk on the beach was as much as I could do, and it did help, but then, as my fitness improved, this wasn't a fitness challenge anymore and 4-5 hours walking just gave me back pain and dehydration.

It's about finding the right program for you.

If you have joint issues or are finding it difficult to move due to your weight, swimming and water exercise is fantastic – there are lots of reasons why working out in water is better than working out on land for many of us. (I'm also a qualified aqua instructor and, when you do the training, learning all the benefits is mind blowing!)

Hydrotherapy or aqua therapy is also fantastic for so many people with serious disabilities, especially if you have access to the right support (and appropriately heated pool!) After all my exploration into healing, visiting spas around the world, I wish everyone had access to the right kind of spa for them. I mean it would be so much cheaper for our society than all the drugs and medical intervention – but here we are, ho hum.

But the most important thing I have found in my life, is to do the exercise you enjoy. You have more chance of keeping up your program and you will also benefit from more mood boosting hormones. A great yoga teacher of mine, Gurmukh once said, 'If you sweat and you smile, that's what makes you happy, healthy and whole.'

Be honest with yourself – when it gets easy – move up a level, work out a little bit harder, or try something new. I'll always remember when a guy I knew came to my class (he was trying to impress me with his fitness because he wanted me to go out with him – apologies to him for sharing this, but it's a teachable moment). This chap was really fit, he went to the gym, he ran 10ks, that kind of thing. When I walked into the hall, he was already running sprints around the floor.

'What are you doing?'

'Warming up.'

'Don't worry, I'll warm you up.' (I'll warm you up good, I was thinking, because a running or sprint warm up was just not going to prepare him for my class, which was in fact, the easiest Zumba class I taught each week, only 45 minutes and my most gentle choreography.)

As soon as we'd warmed up and were getting onto the main workout, he was exhausted. Although he was really fit in terms of running, there were so many muscles in his body that had never tried to salsa or merengue or tango before.

I don't stop between songs, but there is usually a pause of a second or so when I, and a lot of people, grab a glug of water. Each time, he would walk as slowly as possible to the side of the room, sip his water, and then slowly walk back. I've never seen anyone milk a "water break" so much. I would have called him on it, but I could see he was really struggling (and probably regretting the energy he'd used on sprints at the beginning).

It's not just dancing, you can switch to any other kind of activity or sport to give yourself a challenge, but there have been brilliant stories about football and American football teams who have upped their training by doing ballet or Zumba classes. The great thing about dancing is that there's always another type of try – African dance alone probably has more moves than anyone could master in a lifetime. At the moment, I'm using the Zumba Instructor classes I have access to online as part of my Zumba membership – I have over 30 different ones and each time there's something that pushes me to the limit.

Don't be afraid to try things that are a challenge for you. In the NHS advice on how to manage and recover from dizziness, they recommend ballroom dancing, because the rotation helps train us to handle motion without getting dizzy.

In Zumba Gold, we don't take out turns, because they become more difficult for a lot of people as they get older, we do them slower, so you can still do them and you can also get better at turning when you need to in life, without getting dizzy (plus it's fun to turn!)

The same thing with balance – we do moves that act as balance challenges, so although it's scary at first, your balance improves – and is often better than that of younger participants who aren't regularly doing balance challenges.

Let's look at this HIIT concept (that includes the Sprint Training) and I'll explain what I've figured out and my guesswork on why it works so well to increase insulin sensitivity.

High Intensity Interval Training is often a label given to a class in a gym, but it can be used for any kind of exercise where you are working at an intense level, followed by a period of recovery at a lower intensity.

I can tell you, after surgery, when the physio said I had to get out of bed, that was some high intensity sh*t. Also the next night, when the epidural failed and I had to get the nurse to help me out of bed into the chair to try and get it working again… don't give me Mount Everest… that was epic. There is no way on this earth I could have done more than those feats of strength – nothing I do in Zumba is anything like as tough as that (although sometimes the muscle stiffness I have afterwards can give it a run for its money).

Just because a class in a gym is or isn't labelled high intensity that does not mean it will be high intensity (or that the lower intensity intervals will feel like low intensity) for you.

What I love about Zumba is that all the different moves mean that I am usually challenged by about half of them (especially, for some reason, at the moment, the arm movements). I can feel muscles that haven't moved in a particular way for a while or with that oomph shouting out, 'Oh yes, this is high intensity.'

To put it another way, HIIT is a workout where you think, "This is boring," and then a few minutes later, "I can't do it, it's too hard." That's about the right level.

HIIT doesn't have to be Zumba, it could be any sport or exercise as long as it feels intense and also that you get breaks in between the intense training – because as we'll see in a moment, it could be the breaks, the low intensity that is just as important as the high intensity.

I think that what the experts mean when they say HIIT – high intensity intervals with low intensity overall workout is this:

- Aerobic exercise, interspersed with
- Anaerobic bursts of exercise.

Let's look at what this means.

- Aerobic is using oxygen, as we would generally do for a gentle walk, all the way up to someone like Mo Farah running long distances or marathons.
- Anaerobic is without oxygen, not because we are holding our breath, but because the need for energy is so fast, so intense, that we have to use another way of getting that energy super fast to the muscles, like Usain Bolt running the 100 metres.

If you watch the 100 metres you might notice that the athletes don't even seem to breathe or breathe hard (it's only 10 seconds or so).

Essentially, we have two ways of generating energy in the body – aerobic and anaerobic. Without going into too much detail, it makes sense if we have a metabolic problem – a problem with energy and the way our body handles it or rather the sugar that we use to power our body, to exercise both types of metabolism, just as it made sense, when I was rehabbing from an abdominal injury to use belly dancing to get me that abdominal strength and ability back.

Also, according to the American Diabetes Association, when we work aerobically, blood sugar can drop as it's channelled to our muscles, but when we do more intense exercise, we use adrenaline, which can increase blood sugar, releasing it from where it is stored in our bodies – so by mixing the two, hopefully we balance blood sugar better during our workout and, as we've seen, improve insulin sensitivity in the long term.

If we want to burn fat in the body, it has to be aerobic exercise. Anaerobic exercise doesn't burn fat, but it does burn the other energy store in our body, glycogen. (Aerobic exercise burns both glycogen and fat). Having said that, as you'll know anytime you've done a sprint or a fast swim, you'll be gasping for breath afterwards and so will continue to exercise aerobically when that sprint is over (our low intensity moment of a HIIT workout).

So my guesswork is this:

- Aerobic exercise helps us to burn fat, and, despite what some so called "expert" websites will tell you, you can also healthily build and tone muscle at an aerobic level (just ask Mo Farah) and we'll also burn glycogen when it makes sense for the body to do so,

- But anaerobic exercise will force us to burn glycogen, which is a more readily available source of energy, and the action of burning it will indicate to the body that we would like more glycogen please, readily available for our muscles to use next time – which means the body will convert what we're eating into glycogen rather than more fat. (That's my theory.)

One thing it is important to remember is that anaerobic exercise burning glycogen is going to release lactic acid into the body - which can lead to that unfortunate soreness after exercise called DOMS (delayed onset muscle soreness). On the one hand, if you get that, you know you're working anaerobically and to a high level of intensity, and also – on the upside as well – your body will get better at handling lactic acid and so you shouldn't suffer from DOMS for too long (give it a couple of weeks) and then you can train even harder and see even more benefits of your workout.

Whatever you are doing, if you want to create your own high intensity interval training (HIIT) all you have to do is work at a low intensity pace (preferably for 10-15 minutes to warm your body up) and then take your movement up to a pace where you are really doing your best – for example, after 10-15 minutes of gentle swimming in the pool, swim for a few minutes or even seconds (remember Usain Bolt runs the 100 metres in less than 10 seconds!) as hard and fast as you can. You can repeat that several times and then make sure at the end, you give yourself time to cool down, moving at a lower intensity for 10-12 minutes again – and stretch!

High Intensity Does NOT Have To Be High Impact

I am a low impact fitness specialist, having trained to teach Zumba Gold® and having taught people in wheelchairs and with disabilities.

High intensity is when we work really hard – technically so hard that we are working anaerobically – our aerobic metabolism just can't keep up with the energy demand, but that doesn't necessarily mean sprinting (and it certainly doesn't mean burpees – I've never done a burpee and I certainly don't think I ever will – it looks like the least fun exercise ever).

High impact is, for example, jumping or running and can be painful, difficult or impossible – and certainly inadvisable for a lot of people – especially people hitting middle age when our bodies start to behave (or misbehave) differently and our ability to recover from high impact exercise changes.

You can absolutely do high intensity exercise without high impact – in fact my Monday morning online class (Zumba Gold®) is exactly that. It is more hard work than a lot of the Zumba classes I've done – even the ones online from Zumba Home Office with the best Zumba Instructors in the world.

How do we make things intense? Especially if we don't want high impact?

Take a quick look at "Strictly Come Dancing" or "Dancing With The Stars" – take a look at the slower dances – the rumba particularly. Look at the effort required to hold a move or move the hips in a certain way. That's difficult and high intensity.

Belly dancing can be fast and frenetic or it can be so slow that your body aches from holding and moving muscles in such a controlled way.

Hold your arms out, if you can, and hold them there for a few seconds. Can you start to feel the effort, the intensity?

What I love about Zumba, and also about swimming, is that you use so many parts of your body. When you swim hard, it is an incredible intensity, when you salsa or merengue, holding in your core muscles, that's a deep tissue workout that is going to pay off (sometimes with a bit of DOMS as well, which isn't as much fun, but hey).

Do not confuse high intensity with high impact, because most of us who are clinically obese may find running and jumping pretty challenging. I certainly didn't do it in the first week, but now… okay, I don't favour the one workout which has soooooo much jumping, but the one I did yesterday had a fair amount – and I found myself doing it, and enjoying it (it definitely helped that the instructor looked pretty overweight himself, I guess I felt that if he could do it, so could I).

In the class I teach each week, we hit high intensity in the warm up, when we are warming up knees and legs with some squats (I know, don't tell me, you LOVE squats!) I've always hated squats (like the vast proportion of people I've taught) and I've found two ways to learn to love them:

1. Use great music. When the music tells you to squat, it doesn't hurt, because it's dancing. "Get Down On It" by Kool & The Gang works wonders!

2. Get good at them. Then it's just showing off ;)

Sometimes people have knee problems or leg problems and find squats too difficult. That's okay. I always say, if you can't go down, go up. Just do a knee lift, one at a time (otherwise it'll be ridiculously high impact) as high as you can, one at a time – you're still working your knees, getting them warmed up, as well as your legs.

As an expert in fitness for people with disabilities, it is MY JOB to adapt exercise so it suits the individual. I'll do it for you too, if you want to join us. If you want to work with a fitness trainer or teacher, remind them that the workout has to suit you. Sometimes you might have to switch class to one more suitable, but when my class has Zumba Gold® in the description it means it's generally a class for older adults or anyone who needs or wants some adaptation to suit their fitness needs. It can't always be individually tailored, because it's a group class, but usually I can give enough alternatives to make it work.

How To Increase SI Through Healthy Eating

I wanted to keep this as a separate chapter because there is so much focus on healthy eating and losing weight in these kind of conversations and there is no doubt in my mind that it works – but it's slower… so much slower than I feel the changes I made by exercising. What, to me, is so exciting about the way I battled insulin resistance is that it was fast enough for me to defeat the monster, or at least keep migraine at bay long enough to exercise more and escape the chronic situation I was in.

I'm really excited about healthy eating in the long term – as well as rediscovering why so many of the eating changes I made when I was at my worst did me so much good, but that first week it was so important that I threw all my energy into exercising and made healthy eating my second priority.

The secret to increasing insulin sensitivity through eating is, in general, to eat food with a low glycaemic index or, low sugar foods. You can look up any food you want to eat and find out how it rates on the Glycaemic Index (GI). It's not about calories, but about how slowly your body absorbs the sugar or energy from the food, making it less stressful for your body to handle that sugar.

There are some added wrinkles, for example, alcohol can make your blood sugar go up, especially if you're drinking a sugary cocktail, but because the alcohol needs to be processed by the liver, which means that your liver can't help release glucose, it can lead to a drop in blood sugar. It's kind of like the argument on whether to drink coffee or not… one pill makes you smaller, one makes you larger… but which is which?

Back to food, another measure you might want to check out is the Glycaemic Load (GL). Whereas glycaemic index is based on a portion that contains 50g of carbohydrate, the glycaemic load is a little bit more sensible as it's based on an average portion size of the food. So, for example, raisins might have a high GI, but really how many raisins are you going to eat? So raisins are labelled as having a low GL. Whereas potatoes – well, you'll probably eat a reasonable amount of those in a dinner.

Back before I was thinking about insulin, I had already adopted quite a few healthy habits. Because migraines can be triggered by low blood sugar, I had automatically chosen snacks with a low GI and also with high magnesium, as this can help with migraines. Basically I was walking around with a bag of nuts. Because nuts contain fibre, fat and protein, they are slower to be absorbed than many other snacks. Similarly beans, which I was trying to eat more of because of the magnesium, are full of fibre and protein and not as easy for the body to process.

It doesn't mean that you can't or shouldn't eat high GI foods, but by eating them with or after low GI foods, you lower the sugar hit your body would take if you just ate them on their own.

It was this old school thinking about food that I had to remember and put into practice. But none of it was as useful to me before, because I had neither the energy to prepare healthy meals or the ability to eat them when I was feeling nauseous. I was eating a lot of ultra processed foods, which, even though they were vegan, were a sugar fest for my body and kicking up my insulin resistance.

Luckily, chasing the magnesium, I had plenty of low GI foods in my diet – chocolate (surprisingly, yes it's low GI, especially if you have the kind with nuts) popcorn, peas (I seemed to eat a lot of peas) nuts, soy milk, vegan cheese (more on that in a mo) apples and bananas… which all helped to balance out the chips.

When I went to my mum or grandma's house and had a piece of cake, I'd also add a handful of nuts to the plate. (It's really great when it's walnut cake and you add a handful of walnuts.)

My vegan cheese, which I was starting to rethink as it is processed, also contains around 20% coconut oil which, although it's a saturated fat, is being studied as it may help reduce insulin resistance. (Many health professionals also want to reclassify it as, although it's technically a saturated fat, it doesn't affect the body in the same way as other unhealthy saturated fats).

Ginger, which I was taking to help fight migraine, is also known to help with blood sugar and has been clinically shown to lower HbA1c results.

One of the biggest changes I made when I started trying to reduce my insulin resistance (and also lose weight) was to look at my portion sizes. Being so nauseous and having gone through times when I couldn't keep down food for one or two days, I ate a lot when I could, and I didn't ever try to restrict myself if I wanted to eat something yummy (even if it wasn't vegan). But I often put so much on my plate that I was struggling to finish – and I was only clearing my plate to avoid having to locate Tupperware for the leftovers (plus oven chips are not that nice left over). So I started putting half of what I thought I would eat on my plate… that way I could always go back and help myself to more, if I was still hungry. It's amazing how much that small change made me feel so much better.

Intermittent fasting is often discussed at this point, but there are two reasons that I don't fast myself:

1. I find it triggers migraines.
2. The research that has been done seems to have been done with all male participants and certainly not female participants going through menopause, when it might not be such a good idea. There are as many voices encouraging it for perimenopausal women as there are voices warning that it can have an adverse effect on hormones, inflammation and blood sugar.

I think I'll leave it for the moment!

Side Effects

You will put on weight rather than lose it to begin with

The first thing that will happen is that your muscles will start to get bigger and stronger. That's great, but muscle weighs more than fat, so don't expect to get on the scales and have quickly lost weight. In fact, I would strongly recommend that you switch to a trouser test – find a pair of trousers or a skirt that you can just about fasten or can't quite fasten and use this or those as a measure of how you're doing. It might take a couple of weeks to see results, but when the effects of all the exercise kick in, you will be amazed at how your body feels.

Then your knickers will fall down!

Yes, also check your underwear and other clothes fit properly before you run for the bus!

You may have detox headaches for the first week or so

As you burn fat as a result of anaerobic exercise, your body will release toxins into the blood stream. Drink lots of fluids and hopefully, as healthy eating becomes easier to do, you will have less toxins to flush out. To be honest, it's hard to separate this out from triggering migraine activity, but I found it was a lot like caffeine withdrawal – only painful for about a week.

You will often get painful DOMS

"Feeling your muscles ache or stiffen for a few days after exercise is normal and is known as delayed onset muscle soreness (DOMS). It can affect people of all fitness levels, particularly after

trying a new activity or pushing yourself a bit harder than usual."
NHS website

There is still a lot we don't know about DOMS, there are many theories for why we get it and how to alleviate it. I'm going to go with the popular theory that it is due to a build up of lactic acid in the muscles, mainly because the best way of getting rid of it is to exercise again.

The best way of avoiding it is to build up exercise slowly, at least for a few days. I didn't do that as, although I knew it would be painful for a few days, honestly nothing for me is as painful or disruptive as migraine, so I made the choice to go hard. You don't have to do that, but, as I've shared, it's the high intensity that really accelerates the increase of insulin sensitivity, so it's up to you how much you want to risk that burning DOMS feeling. If the theory that the cause is a build up of lactic acid, it also means that you are working at an anaerobic (high intensity) level and your body is also learning (or remembering) how to work better anaerobically, so your ability to clear lactic acid you generate in the future should be quicker and less painful.

My experience is that often stopping for an hour or so after a work out, having lots of fluid and a rest can be very beneficial for preventing DOMS – as can taking time in the shower for a massage of affected muscles.

Your belly fat will become more pronounced

Say what!! I often say that we all have a six pack, it's just for a lot of us there's a lot of belly fat on top. When you start to work out, especially those abdominal muscles, whether you're swimming, belly dancing or anything where your core muscles are working, that six pack is going to tighten up and tone – and your belly fat will seem to be more pronounced because it's sitting on top of the muscle. (That's my less than technical way of describing it.) Don't worry – it's part of the process. The more you use your abdominal muscles, the more that fat will get burned up, it often happens quicker than you think and then suddenly… ooh, there's the six pack.

You will have much more laundry

Sorry – but that sweaty gear needs washing. Suddenly you might feel like you're living with a football team that needs its kit washed every week!

You may get more hot flushes initially

If you are perimenopausal or menopausal, you may find that you get more hot flushes – this may be to do with your body circulation improving, or it may also relate to healthy eating.

It's infuriating! that we still don't know why women have hot flushes in perimenopause and menopause (NEWS FLASH – I've figured it out – check out the chapter on hot flushes – it's revolutionary! And it explains why we may get more of them as we do more exercise!) We know there are some things that make them worse, like spicy food, and (no shit, Sherlock) having your bedroom too warm, but I find, even with taking vitamins and having a borderline Arctic bedroom that the hot flushes still plague me.

I did find advice that said they affect overweight and obese women more, turns out that's not actually true – yet another internet urban myth.

I have found that eating beans and peas at night seems to lead to more hot flushes, perhaps because they are high in protein and require more fluid to process (likewise exercising later in the day can lead to more hot flushes as you may not have had the chance to rehydrate or your body is still recovering from exercise which can involve some temperature changes, especially in the muscles). I've found that switching to eating beans and peas at lunchtime and then, in the evening, more water rich foods like fruit and vegetables can help. Basically, treat hot flushes as a symptom of dehydration and treat with fluids and electrolytes such as potassium, sodium and magnesium – bananas are a particularly good post workout snack.

Do I sound like a complete freak if I say that I have started making spring green chips with sea salt as a tasty snack? Just cut up the greens into big squares, cover in oil and leave in the oven for 5-10 minutes. (I usually do these if I've been oven roasting other vegetables, so just throw them in on top and use the oil already in the pan.)

You may injure yourself or already have physical issues or injuries

Starting exercising, especially high intensity, can cause injury. The best way to avoid this, especially if, like me, you're a person of a certain age, is to warm up properly. It drives me nuts how many "fitness professionals" jump into exercise without doing a proper warm up – I'm going to release some more videos on Zumba.com with my own gentle warm ups, but I find particularly the shoulders and arms don't get enough of a warm up in a lot of classes.

A safe way to warm up your shoulders is just by rolling the shoulders back. It's very easy and a little boring, which is why so many instructors don't include it, they're too worried about boring their participants. I'd rather bore my class than have them injured (and I can say, a bit proudly, that the only people – or rather person – to ever get injured in my class was me!) If you're doing a class, or a video at home and you are following someone who is getting a bit too ambitious with arms and shoulders in the warm up – the first 10-15 minutes, just switch in some gentle shoulder rolls until you feel properly warmed up. Keep your arms low (below shoulder) until you're warmed up, feel ready, or unless you are just doing some easy stretches to the ceiling (I would also do these in the first five minutes).

Take it easy, you can always build intensity when you've done a move small or slow a couple of times.

We all get carried away at times, and if you do feel that you have an injury, treat it depending on the severity. (Ask your instructor if you're working out in person). If it's a strain or a sprain then RICE – Rest, Ice, Comfortable Support and Elevate. If it's more severe, get professional support – preferably a physiotherapist.

"By 2024, all adults in England will to be able to see a

musculoskeletal first contact physiotherapist at their local GP practice without being referred by a GP." NHS website

If at all possible, don't ditch your next workout because of a minor injury, remember what you are working towards. I've worked with people at all levels of health and fitness and while we might not want to work out because of a problem or a minor injury, if we don't, we are building up trouble in our general health – whether it's heart disease or insulin resistance. If you have a shoulder injury, work out the rest of your body. If there are a few moves you can't do, don't do them. But in the words of Martin Luther King Jr. "If you can't fly then run, if you can't run then walk, if you can't walk then crawl, but whatever you do you have to keep moving forward."

If you have a particular health problem, look around for classes for people with similar issues – or for a Zumba Gold® Instructor who is trained to adapt a class to your needs.

It drives me nuts how many people I've worked with who have told me they have been turned away by gyms because they've got an underlying health condition. That's like a doctor turning you away because you're too sick. Fine, if you can't help someone, but call an ambulance – or help them find the right class for them. The only time we should be saying, 'No,' to someone is when the doctor has told them not to exercise (or if they're trying to do the wrong class for them – i.e. kids and adults have different exercise needs).

Magnesium and B2

B2 and magnesium are two supplements that are recommended as a first step in treating migraine patients, partly because these two supplements are rather effective and also cause little to no side effects except in very rare instances. (Apart from B2 making your pee bright yellow and magnesium supplements giving you diarrhoea.)

They both have a very high rate of improving or preventing migraine.

Magnesium is recommended at a dose of 400mg for migraine sufferers. And if that doesn't work, go up to 600mg. The big drawback of magnesium supplements is the diarrhoea – so I've been following a regimen of getting 400 or 600mg through diet, and only topping up with 100mg of magnesium in my daily Menopace tablet and the occasional small tablet, 187.5mg, when migraines stop me from eating enough.

Magnesium has also been shown to be really effective at improving insulin sensitivity. A dose of 300mg is recommended to help people who are on the path to type 2 diabetes.

What does magnesium do and why does it affect insulin sensitivity?

Well, it has so many functions within the body I couldn't list them all, but one important thing that magnesium does it to improve the communication between cells, allowing insulin to work more effectively and to store energy in cells (that glucose uptake) quicker.

So again, I wonder if this is another indication that migraine is more related to insulin sensitivity than we know – or at least we communicate to migraine sufferers? I mean, if I had known this before…

B2 or riboflavin is recommended at a dose of 400mg for migraine sufferers, which is around 300 times the average daily recommended dose. The role of B2 in the body is to help convert food into energy as well as supporting other enzymes in the body. I've found it to be very effective at helping me to keep migraines at bay, and at times, when a migraine is threatening, I find taking it can be preventative within a few minutes. Again, this leads me to wonder if there is more to the possibility that migraine is much more related to metabolism, to the movement of food to energy, or blood sugar to stored energy, than we have realised before.

If you want to increase B2 and magnesium in your body, then a healthy diet should do it. For migraine sufferers, getting 400mg of B2 is probably only feasible through tablets. I once worked out that to get the right amount of B2 (remember, it's 300 x what normal people are recommended to need) I'd have to eat around 40kg of red grapes a day.

The best thing (and probably the reason my HbA1c was so good) was, by trying to eat more magnesium, I was including in my

diet a lot of things that are great for improving insulin sensitivity –
nuts, beans, soy milk, tofu, popcorn, dark chocolate, wholemeal
bread, Marmite, cacao, spinach and other fruit and vegetables.

It made sense that when I started on the B2 and also on the
magnesium that my migraines eased off, but it wasn't enough to stop
the monster in its tracks.

Physiotherapy

If you need help to get moving because of an underlying problem, just remember that GP surgeries have a deadline!

"By 2024, all adults in England will to be able to see a musculoskeletal first contact physiotherapist at their local GP practice without being referred by a GP." NHS website

So if you do have a problem, or if exercising aggravates or causes an injury, please do call your GP surgery and ask to see a physiotherapist.

It's All About the Dosage

If we treat exercise as we would a medication, say for migraine, we'd do it every day for at least three weeks before we'd decide whether it was having any impact.

We'd start on whatever we thought was the appropriate dosage, and then increase or decrease depending on how easy or difficult we were finding it to take, or how effective we felt it was.

Instead, what we often do with exercise is to "give it a go" for a few days and then let something get in the way – other commitments, work, maybe we run out of clean sportswear, maybe the weather is bad or someone is having a party, maybe we get DOMS or we have a minor injury. But if we stop and think how important it is, and the difference it can make to our health, I think we'd make it a top priority.

I've made exercising for an hour a priority for years. The times when I didn't do it were often when I was feeling better, when I had a lot to do for my family, when they were unwell. It wasn't long before I was unwell too. I guess that's something I have in common with many carers. What I've learned (and really relearned) these last few weeks, is that when I make a certain dosage of exercise (this time 45 minutes to one hour of Zumba) my top priority, it's not long before I can do way more for my family (and way more work and everything else) than I could have done a few weeks before. Just by changing the way I looked at exercise, to making it like rehab – utterly essential for the rest of my life - I've overcome the lurking monster that was costing me so much of my life and so much of my quality of life.

If exercise was a pill, we'd all be on it.

If I had known the difference this was going to make, I would have started it years ago.

There's an old Japanese adage: "To fall down seven times and get up eight." I've often used it, every time I have to get back up from a migraine, and I know this exercise regime is going to get interrupted – when I get sick, from migraine or anything else – but if I can get back up from the kind of migraines I've suffered in the last few years, I know I can keep getting up.

How To Exercise When You Can't Exercise

I've spoken before about having to rehab from surgery and other injuries. I know how impossible it can seem.

Please don't forget that before I started this exercise program, I had already made a commitment to exercising for an hour a day, even if it was only a walk round the village. If I couldn't do an hour, I would do twenty minutes, if not twenty minutes, then just around the living room.

Even now, there are days when I try to do a little more and set out to walk to the corner of the lane – five minutes away – and sometimes I can't even do that. Yesterday, I had a migraine and did nothing more than get out of bed for cups of tea and a few slices of toast. What I've learned from this research is that it takes three days of inactivity for me to start to lose the insulin sensitivity I've built up. That's great for those days when it is actually impossible for me to exercise. This morning I got up and did a gentle workout, but I'm taking it easy for the rest of the day.

The first thing is to make exercise a priority. When I had my last intense physio sessions (around about 2010) my physio would work me to the point of collapse, and then I would get on the Tube and walk home. When I first really put my back out, I would hobble about five minutes down the road to see the physio, who would massage and help me through my exercise and then I would hobble back to bed. It's really hard to commit to an hour, or five minutes of exercise, when we know it's going to cost us our whole day's energy

– but that is rehab. Sometimes it's the only thing we can do. But in the same way as an alcoholic or drug addict may have to commit to 28 days in a facility to have the best chance to beat their illness, perhaps we too have to commit 28 days to doing something that will give us a chance at having a life, at staying alive.

Having a migraine condition, people often look at me as if I'm normal. When I stagger down the road, trying to get moving, with my dark glasses on, I always feel like people will judge me as being hungover. Sometimes I worry that my neighbours will think that I'm an alcoholic or a drug addict, sometimes I want a T-shirt that says, 'I have a migraine', especially when I have to move away from someone on the bus because their perfume (to me) reeks to high heaven, when someone on their phone makes me want to throttle them, when my mum calls me with the TV on in the background and I have to ask her, for the millionth time, to turn it off. I sit in the disabled seats at the front of the bus (unless someone else more in need gets on) because I'm now prone to motion sickness unless I can see the road ahead. I've thought about getting one of those sunflower badges to show I have a hidden disability (but I don't think I'm actually allowed - I haven't yet been officially classified as disabled).

It's been my wish for years to be healthy again.

Isn't it worth 100% commitment, doing my best, you doing your best, for the chance at being, if not completely healthy, then healthier?

Take a day off from everything… except exercise. What

would that look like for you?

The big wake up call for me was my sight. I thought I could run up this debt, putting on weight, eating badly, because I knew how to rehab my body when this phase of my life was done. But then my eyesight was threatened.

Another wake up call was realising that I could damage my kidneys. My brother had to be on dialysis for years. It's a life saving treatment, but one I wouldn't wish on anyone. As good as it is, being on dialysis means getting progressively weaker, sicker as there are some things that dialysis can't handle.

Insulin resistance can lead to type 2 diabetes. Within 3-5 years this can cause kidney damage. Diabetic patients are often dialysis patients. I'll do everything I can to avoid being either.

If you have cancer and someone tells you that chemotherapy could save your life, most people would do it, because it's a chance to live.

But we ignore the warnings to exercise and eat healthier, because we don't realise how important they are and to be honest, they're not loud enough, not strong enough. We need to act on the smoke alarm – not when the fire engines are showing up!

All we have to do, all you have to do, is your best.

HIIT That Monster!

There is something just wonderful about feeling that I am fighting migraine when I am exercising. Every time there is a moment in a song when there is some kicking or punching, I am kicking or punching migraine!

After all these years of suffering, especially the last few, I have finally found a way to fight, to HIIT back! It feels great.

It feels like that moment when the townspeople get their mojo back, when the monster is injured and they all, even the kids, even the old ladies, pick up a bit of wood, a pole and get ready to lamp the thing (or should that be Thing).

When you get clear on what you are doing, if this works for you and your migraines, then use that energy, that frustration, because, okay, you can never pay migraine back, can you? But at least it feels like you can get a few good punches in.

Over Training

Having been a professional fitness instructor and having taught way too many classes at times, I've definitely overdone it, overworking my body, but I hope I haven't drifted into starving my body of the energy it needed. I want to explain this, just as a warning, if you find you go a bit too far with your fitness and even when your healthy eating becomes unhealthy.

You have to remember that even Olympic athletes do not maintain "peak" fitness outside of their competing seasons. It's unhealthy to do that. People who train to run the 100 metres as fast as a human being can are always courting disaster – at that level of "fitness", injuries are more likely. You may look at the professional dancers on "Strictly Come Dancing" but many of them, no matter how fit they look, are using their time off for necessary surgery – for knees, ligaments and other parts of bodies that were never meant to work so hard.

Our peak fitness is the level at which we are the healthiest, when we are not taxing our internal organs or glands – like the adrenals which create adrenaline.

You can feel it in your body, when you're overworking and too much adrenaline can cause forgetfulness among other things.

As for starvation or what we could call "ketosis", we often hear this term for diets where carbs are restricted, causing the body to burn fat and even protein for energy. I've always lost weight as part of a high carb diet – those carbs being fruit and vegetables which, as well as being great sources of energy, also have so many other healthy things inside them – not least magnesium.

For some professional fitness instructors, we talk about "ketosis" as being when we start to burn our own muscles for energy – when we're just not eating enough to sustain the energy expenditure of our classes.

Ideally, when we're losing excess weight, especially when we're obese, we are not eating enough to compensate for the energy we're burning – that's why we lose weight but, first and foremost, we're building a healthy body, we're building stores of easily accessible energy so we feel energetic and not fatigued, so we can do what we want.

Restricting carbohydrates can have very unfortunate side effects – like damage to internal organs, especially kidneys – something that is just not in our best interests.

By eating healthily and exercising at the best level for us, and reducing insulin resistance, we're getting our bodies back to where they ought to be – ready, willing and able to have fun - not dragging because of too much food, too little exercise or vice versa.

Once we hit a healthy weight, we need to make sure that we ARE eating enough to compensate for the energy we're burning, especially if we want to continue to build and maintain muscle.

Safety first!

(A little cautionary tale about weight loss. When I went to give my brother a kidney, I was at the heaviest weight I could be and still be deemed healthy enough to do it. I was working out every day in the gym – I'd never been healthier.

Although I maintained a lot of that fitness after the surgery – including being able to touch my toes! - my body changed dramatically as it tried to recover from the surgery and rebuild all the damage. I lost a stone within a few days and I lost the majority of my muscle mass as my body "cannibalised" it in order to rebuild the tissues damaged by the surgery.)

The body will "take what it needs" and if it needs protein to rebuild tissue, and we do not or cannot eat protein, it will strip down muscle in order to do the job.

If it needs energy to survive, it will strip down muscle when there is no carbohydrate store available. Think of it like the poor widow in a house who starts to burn the furniture for heat because there is no firewood left. We do not want that.

Sometimes it feels as though we are at odds with our body, it can feel scary when it does things that we don't understand or don't think we want, but a lot of this process is about understanding where we have not been serving our body, taking care of it, even if that lack of care was because we just did not understand what was in our beautiful body's best interests, or because we just, whether because of health, Covid, caring or other life circumstances, couldn't.

Ancient HIIT

My business, Pearl Escapes, started with the premise of discovering all the wonderful things in the world and sharing them with people, especially massage and spa treatments because, when I discovered proper massage in Morocco, it made such an instant difference to me – it was healing.

In 2019, I published my latest guide to healing which had around 500 types. While I'd been researching, I'd discovered that so much of what we need is available in ancient indigenous healing, from the massage to the pilgrimages, the answer to so many of our cries for help lay not in the modern medicine but in our ancient lineages. (And so much of our modern medicine also draws from these lineages.)

When we question our diet and look back, we realise how much of our modern diet causes our illness – ultra processed foods and refined sugar.

When I was recovering from the kidney donation surgery, it was belly dancing that gave me back the full use of my hips and pelvis. It was reiki that gave me back the feeling in my scarred abdomen (five years after the surgery).

If we look clearly, we can see that we used to have a HIIT practice since the time we began dancing.

Zumba works because it's based on world rhythms – African music, South American movement, belly dancing which has been used for generations to support women getting ready to give birth, to recover and perhaps even during perimenopause – perhaps if I had kept up with the belly dancing, I wouldn't have gotten myself into this situation! It certainly one of the best things we can do to avoid having a hip replacement later in life.

Scottish dancing, Russian dancing, Native American music and movement… when I travelled to South East Asia, to Borneo, I witnessed so many incredible styles of dance coming from the different peoples of Borneo.

Like eating a diet that is based on more fruit and vegetables, that includes things like ginger and naturally high levels of magnesium, our cultural dances have always held the secret to keeping us healthy, to keeping our monsters at bay.

The Role of Hot Flushes and Cold Nights

Sometimes it's hard to figure out what's a good thing and what's a bad thing, especially when we're talking about biology, and life.

Migraines are bad. But when I look at my life, I see that they've often acted as an early warning system, something that's kicked in when I'm trying to live my life putting up with awful jobs, terrible relationships. They've led to me quitting more than one job. When I look at my life today, despite all the negatives, what is great is that I have created a life that allows me as much heaven as my health will allow. My home works around me, supporting me and, as my migraines get better, I see how easy it is for me to take on too much, put other people's needs always before my own and not find that time to sit in the sun. I need to remember, as I hopefully get better, just what I love about life and what's important – because migraines have, above all things, given me the gift of perspective and consciousness of what is important, just as people who have experienced other health issues and crises have found truth.

After finding so many answers by looking deeper at insulin resistance and migraine traits, I thought I would turn my attention to hot flushes or flashes, especially after my doctor told me, 'We don't know why hot flushes occur.' They've been getting progressively worse for me, particularly since I started exercising more and since the weather has got colder.

(Some of those of you who are keen eyed might have also noted that night sweats are also a symptom of hypoglycaemia in diabetic patients – could the hot flushes and night sweats be a symptom of very slight low blood sugar at night?)

Instinctively, I decided to look at a mysterious substance in the human body which, I remember from my Biology "A" Level, is responsible for generating heat and is found more in people who are *less* obese – brown adipose tissue (BAT) – or brown fat (and, it's been said, can also be increased or activated by more exercise).

BAT is the reason that we mammals are so successful because, unlike other animals, it allows us to generate heat without moving, or shivering, or sitting in the sun. It's called thermogenesis. And it's been shown to be regulated by oestrogen. ("Estradiol Regulates Brown Adipose Tissue Thermogenesis via Hypothalamic AMPK" Pablo B. Martínez de Morentin et al, 2014.)

It turns out that this is quite the hot topic, especially when it comes to obesity, type 2 diabetes and weight loss. And… there's even been a recent study, the first study into BAT and hot flushes conducted by Dr. Lynnette Leidy Sievert and Dr. Daniel E. Brown presented at the 2023 Annual Meeting of The Menopause Society which asked, "Can You Actually Have a Hot Flash in Cold Weather?" (yes, I can tell them, yes, you can, oh, so many, many hot flashes) which concluded that:

"…an increase in BAT activity almost tripled the likelihood

of hot flashes, one of the most commonly reported menopause-related symptoms…"

"…in addition to considering the role of BAT in lipid and glucose metabolism, diabetes and obesity, additional research is required to further examine the role of BAT in relation to hot flashes, especially in cool ambient temperatures…"

What makes this such a hot (oh, why is everything so hot?) topic is that scientists are starting to discover a lot more about the relationship between white and brown fat and how they work to prevent or create obesity and type 2 diabetes.

What we call white fat (or just fat for those of us who have a lot of it) also known as white adipose tissue (WAT) primarily stores energy for us, but has also been shown to produce a whole host of chemicals and hormones. (These include the mysterious leptin which was thought, when discovered, to be the cure for obesity, hence its name from the Greek *leptos* – thin. That was 28 years ago and it turned out, not so much the cure for obesity. Another important chemical produced by white adipose tissue is resistin, a protein that is reported to induce insulin resistance, which is another reason we are more at risk of developing insulin resistance when we have more white adipose tissue.)

The healthier we are, in general, the more BAT we will have in relation to WAT – it's all about balance.

When we get cold, especially when we get progressively

cold, as in the temperature drops gradually, our BAT gets better at producing heat to keep us warm. At least one of the studies (the one by Cohen and Spiegelman which I'll get onto in a moment) has estimated that this could burn between 25 and 400 calories a day. (Or in my case, about 4,000 each night!)

But there are two more (kinda) types of fat:

- BAT that has whitened. Another thing that happens when we become obese (that's me too), is that our brown adipose tissue converts into tissue similar to white fat, and both types of tissue become dysfunctional and inflamed. One of the reasons for this "death" of brown fat is high ambient temperature. ("Brown adipose tissue whitening leads to brown adipocyte death and adipose tissue inflammation" Petra Kotzbeck et al, 2018.)

- Beige fat cells which exist in white fat cells and act like them, unless it gets cold and then they act like brown fat cells, generating heat. "Brown and Beige Fat: Molecular Parts of a Thermogenic Machine" by Paul Cohen and Bruce M Spiegelman, 2015

A lot of research on BAT is about the relationship between it, WAT and obesity – researchers are hoping to unlock the secrets of how they work together and the many other functions of white fat and the hormones and other chemicals it secretes. Our white fat can be considered the largest "gland" or endocrine tissue in the human body, just as our skin is actually the largest organ.

One thing we can consider is that the time a lot of these hormones are active is in the early hours of the morning and my hot flushes are craziest between around 1am and 5am. (What complicates things is that a lot of the research into BAT and perhaps more importantly its relationship with WAT has been derived from animal studies – mice and rats – which, like us, are mammals, but critically (especially for us hot flush sufferers) are nocturnal animals – so I don't think this is something we can learn from them.)

Okay, so, there's still so much we don't know, but we do know that hot flushes cause us to turn down the ambient temperature – the thermostat – because they make you feel like you're in a sauna! (Or like a dream I had last week, in a hot tub in a fur coat.)

So turning down the heat will help protect our brown adipose tissue, and… "Since cold robustly activates brown and beige fat, some investigators have suggested that moderate cold exposure could be used as a therapeutic approach. At least in healthy subjects, daily exposure to 19°C for 2 hours was sufficient to activate brown fat, resulting in weight loss. In another small human study, alternating cycles of cold exposure were shown to result in improved insulin sensitivity. While these studies suggest the potential of cold as a treatment modality, our societal preference for thermal comfort may make this unfeasible as a broad approach." "Brown and Beige Fat: Molecular Parts of a Thermogenic Machine" by Paul Cohen and Bruce M Spiegelman, 2015

19 degrees? My bedroom hasn't seen 19 degrees since the summer. Last night's attempt to sleep was a new low of 15.5 – a night of being both hot and cold all night, but more sleep than the night before. (Although this could also answer why my migraines get so much worse during the summer and hot nights, because my insulin resistance may have gone up…)

We do know that hot flushes are more common when our BAT is active… which happens when the temperature is low… so although generating heat is burning calories and moving me further away from obesity and insulin resistance… could it be that progressively turning down the temperature is actually causing, instead of helping my hot flushes?

Wow.

So the other big question, which I haven't been able to find the answer to is this, "Do hot flushes damage brown adipose tissue or are they a way of protecting it?"

I just don't think we've looked yet.

But I'm going to speculate. I'm going to speculate that, like DOMS, the increased hot flushes are an indication that I'm going in the right direction with exercise, that I'm creating more brown adipose tissue and preventing it from deteriorating into more white fat (which I certainly do not need!)

They are a way of pushing women in perimenopause to turn

down the thermostat and certainly not wrap up too warm at night, which protects brown adipose tissue.

Perhaps they are part of us women going through perimenopause and menopause adjusting to a new, lower core temperature as our oestrogen drops?

Perhaps, like fat, there are at least two types of hot flush or night sweat. The kind where we are actually warm and need to cool down (possibly accompanied by sweating – luckily I don't sweat at night) and the kind that occur because our BAT is becoming more active – possibly because we are exposing ourselves to colder and colder temperatures, which is a natural response to hot flushes which are a natural way for our body to protect us from insulin resistance and obesity as we go through perimenopause and menopause.

But perhaps it's okay for me just to be cold or cool during the day, protecting my brown (and beige) fat and maybe I can give myself a break at night by not turning the thermostat down quite so cold?

I can't wait to try it tonight!

It worked! So beautifully! I was toastie warm and had only two or three "bothersome" hot flushes – nothing like what I've been experiencing. I think there really are two types of hot flushes! It's time to write it all down clearly:

Pearl Howie's Hot Flash Theory

There are two kinds of hot flush or flash.

The first is what scientists recognise as VMS which stands for Vasomotor Symptoms – this is where we are too warm and, as a response, our blood vessels dilate, causing us often to go bright red (in the middle of the night I look like a tomato). It's like blushing, but extreme. It can also include sweating. Common literature suggests that these type of hot flushes last very briefly (usually because we kick off the covers, turn on the fan and turn down the heat, or open the window).

The second kind is what I have been experiencing recently: a much more intense, long lasting, burning feeling that comes from deep within and, crucially, occurs when I am cold. My theory is that this kind of hot flash is caused by brown or beige adipose tissue (BAT) generating heat (thermogenesis) in order to warm up my core temperature. But because this is a new phenomenon in my body, it overheats, then triggering a VMS hot flush and causing a kind of yo-yo-ing, always too hot or cold and rarely comfortable at night.

This kind of hot flush can occur every few hours or several times an hour and it lasts for minutes, rather than seconds.

This type of hot flash DOES burn calories and it does keep our brown and beige adipose tissue active, which helps to prevent obesity and insulin resistance, in many ways that we don't understand, but certainly by maintaining the balance between white and brown fat and preventing inflammation and dysfunction of both.

At a certain level (before the sleep torture and dehydration) hot flashes are GOOD for us!

Why does it happen in the first place?

"The change" or menopause is a woman's body (generally) going from one which can grow, feed and nurture a baby and infants to one which does not. White fat helps us stay warm by insulating, but women being comfortable at the same temperature as is safest for a baby (we estimate 19 degrees Centigrade) would help them to keep babies and infants safe (and warm).

After this time, a woman's health is probably best served by heat functions (and let's not forget that, before we developed so many heating solutions, staying warm, like storing energy, was an essential part of staying alive) that are more like a man's and certain studies have shown that men are more likely to generate heat from brown adipose tissue when necessary, helping them to survive at lower temperatures.

We are starting to understand that being at lower temperatures encourages not just the preservation of brown and beige fat, but can also increase and activate it.

In practical terms, what does this mean?

While women suffering from hot flashes should keep their bedrooms cool, they shouldn't go overboard (like me!) and drop the temperature so far that BAT has to go into overdrive to keep them warm (and then too warm) at night. If they do make this mistake, the upside is that they are burning calories and increasing insulin sensitivity.

Cold exposure is still great for the body in terms of preventing obesity and insulin resistance, but we can also do this during the day, as the previous study showed that as little as two hours at temperatures less than 19 degrees Centigrade is beneficial (which is as warm as I'd ever want to be) and we can finally get some sleep at night!

P.S. We can also look at the reasons men get hot flashes. Although the focus tends to be around testosterone levels (because medicine and sports tend to be biased about testosterone levels) which, like oestrogen levels dropping, can cause us to have hot flashes, again, no one knows how or why.

We do know that hot flashes can also occur in men who are obese, have type 2 diabetes, or when they experience stress and anxiety… or lack of sleep – all things which affect insulin sensitivity.

Although we don't yet know the secrets of brown adipose tissue, white (and whitened and beige) fat, we do know that it is intricately linked with obesity.

So we could again surmise that these hot flashes in men are doing the same thing as they are doing in women – helping us to protect our brown adipose tissue, our ability to generate heat when needed for survival and improving our insulin sensitivity.

In the End

Maybe I'm wrong.

No matter how scientific we are, or careful with our assumptions, we make mistakes. Doctors make mistakes.

Maybe this is all just a coincidence and my migraines have eased off at exactly the same time as I started intense exercise.

Maybe it works, but only for *my* monster.

Or maybe this could be a turning point, for everyone who is suffering so much from migraine.

What I do know is this: One of the UK's top neurologists, when talking about migraine, said, 'It does go, maybe in your 60s, 70s, 80s, or 90s, but it robs you of some of the best years of your life.' I feel like that, have felt like that for the last few years. After losing time to Covid, I was losing years of my life – perhaps another 7-10 years, to migraine. People get less time for some pretty awful crimes.

But I'll tell you what migraine has also robbed me of in the last few years – health, fitness, being able to fit into my clothes, being able to eat healthily, being able to enjoy getting sweaty, and if I'd let it carry on, who knows what it might have robbed me of… my eyesight, my kidney, my beating heart?

So I had a rock bottom moment and I'm getting my insulin sensitivity back, I'm making sure that I don't lose my eyesight, don't lose my kidney, that I have *excellent* cardiovascular health and, I hope that you can use whatever I have shared in this book to get back whatever migraine, or Covid, or perimenopause or any other issue or ill health has tried to take from you.

Use that monster's weakness and in the words of Ripley in "Alien" tell it, "I got you...you son of a b*tch."

The Plan – Step by Step

I want to make this as simple as I can, because, unfortunately, vague directions like "lose weight" and "eat healthily" have gotten us into this mess. As I said before, with medication we are more precise, "take one a day with or before food" or even "take every four hours, up to three times daily," so I want to make this as simple, as step by step as I can.

1.   Choose an exercise.

I chose Zumba because it's worked so well for me in the past (don't forget, I also do a physio/yoga routine of around 5 minutes each day to take care of my back which is prone to injury) and because, as a Zumba Instructor, I have an online library of over 30 workouts and extra exercises at my fingertips, but I've also had great results from belly dancing and general gym workouts in the past.

Choose something you like (or hate the least). My research has focused on HIIT, but aerobic exercise will also work to increase insulin sensitivity, as will weight training and anaerobic exercise (although bear in mind that a good warm up will probably be aerobic, so you will normally get some aerobic exercise as part of your workout).

Choose more than one exercise if you like – I've had great results in the past by aiming for one Zumba session, one swim and one hike each day.

If you are really unable to do any exercise (and trust me, I've been there – still am there on some migraine days) focus on just standing up or gentle walking after you've eaten, as this will help your body deal with the food you've just eaten and may help increase insulin sensitivity. The key is to do as much as you can, as soon as you can. Each day you should be able to do a little more.

## 2.	Make the time.

Start today if possible. As much as we make plans, all we are in control of is the action we take right now, in the present. We can do the preparation – indeed, we need to put on the right clothes, anything else we need for safety, but it's the moment we go that starts the change in our bodies.

If you read my diary, you'll see that I've had false starts, the moments when I tried to slowly increase exercise but, because of my poor health, I needed to attack this monster as quick and as hard as possible. I think it was the moment, after a six day migraine, when I ended up in A&E, and then spent one day supporting my brother for a health thing, then the next accompanying him to a hospital appointment, that I sat in the hospital cafeteria with my mum and my brother and it came out of me, quite loud and abrupt, surprising even me, 'I have to focus on *my* health now.' Of course, they both agreed, because people do, when you say it out loud.

When you have a health problem, especially one that's been going on for a long time, it's tempting to put it off for one more day, because really, what difference does a day make? Well, it's one more day of illness, one more day of pain, one more day of suffering. Or in the case of migraine, it might just be the only day you have to do this, before the monster strikes again.

Caring is my job, and in this moment what I did was to say to my bosses, 'I need some time off.'

If I could have a surgery that would fix migraine (there are a couple of procedures…) would I book a week off in order to have it? You bet I would. A week, to get my life back? Where do I sign?

After a few weeks, I was not only able to go back to caring full time, I was able to do so much more than I had before. This is the case you can make to a boss, to a partner, to your family, if you need to take time off in order to battle insulin resistance and take care of your short and long term health before it deteriorates any further. For me this was rehab, and if your health is such you would take time off for doctor's appointments, for physio, then it makes sense to take the time off to rehab your body yourself.

3.   Consider your dosage and the time you exercise.

Generally, I exercise in the morning, but there were days when I exercised later, because I had some things I needed to do in the morning. If you really need a rest day, take a rest day. Just be honest.

I decided to aim for every day because it's easier and it gave me more of a window to make a difference before my next migraine.

Some studies recommend HIIT at least five times a week.

Crucially, avoid missing more than two days in a row as three days of inactivity are enough to start that move towards insulin resistance again.

Consider that each good session increases your insulin sensitivity for more than 16 hours, so ask yourself if twice a day is necessary (it might work even better for you, who knows?)

Sometimes people talk about accountability and you can definitely team up with someone else, or even post your progress on social media. People can be very supportive. I decided to start writing it down in a diary and to keep a tally of the number of sessions I had done in the previous 7 days, that was my reality check. When I was teaching, I started a reward scheme with printed cards. I would sign the card each time someone did a class and people would get rewards when they did, 5, 10, 20 or even a hundred classes. (People will apparently do a lot for a pair of Zumba socks.) It definitely improved class attendance because people were always looking at their card when I signed it and saying, 'Oh my goodness, I haven't been for a month.' Give yourself a gold star on a chart in the kitchen if you want – you will have deserved it.

4.   Give yourself the best possible chance of success.

Make sure you have eaten something an hour or two before you begin, make sure you are hydrated, that you are wearing shoes (if you're wearing shoes) that are comfortable and supportive. (Weirdly enough, the day before I began in earnest, I decided to walk all over town to get myself moving. I was wearing shoes I'd been wearing all summer but still managed to give myself terrible blisters.)

5.   Warm up properly.

The warm up is crucial to avoiding injury. The last thing you want is to injure yourself and be unable to continue your program. If you are doing a class in a gym or online and you feel that the warm up is too aggressive, just do what feels right to you. Your body will naturally loosen and warm up with easy, gradual movement (especially your arms).

If it feels awful, give yourself 15 minutes for your body to warm up as that's often when you finally have enough oxygenated blood for things to feel easier.

Keep going.

6.   Stretch.

Even if you just go for a long walk, stretching is important to prevent injury.

7.   Allow yourself recovery time.

Rehabbing your body is often painful. Learn the difference between when you have overdone it (muscle spasms and strains) and the natural "hangover" of increased exercise – DOMS, needing to drink more fluids and yes, even eat more often. Feeling tired and needing to take a nap or just sit down more often, even if people look at you funny. The time to take a shower or even a massage or sports massage.

8. **Allow yourself time to deal with the other aspects of increased exercise…**

Laundry, realising your clothes just won't cut it (please don't go and buy lots of new things because you may find you start to lose weight very quickly once you get going – you can always check out charity shops).

9. **Look for signs of areas where you need more support.**

For me, I did my first workout in bare feet and then realised I needed to wear my good workout shoes to support my ankle. I'm okay with my bra tops, but sooner or later, I will probably need to upgrade to one with more support. If you aggravate underlying weaknesses – commonly back problems, ankle problems, things like plantar fasciitis – see a physiotherapist. Remember that, from 2024, everyone in the UK should be able to see a physio at their GP practice without referral. (Should is the operative word – but remember that private physios are not that expensive when compared to good health and you may also be covered if you have a private health plan through work – that's how I got six weeks of physio just before I became a Zumba Instructor. I had to pay for the few times I went back with issues I developed when I started teaching, but it has always been worth it for me whenever I had an injury.)

10.   Start eating healthier.

I think you probably know how. If not, try not to pick up faddy diets, just look up the foods you like and find out which ones are low GI or low GL. I did a strange thing in the supermarket the other day. I really like aubergines, but I think they're too expensive and a bit small! 95p for an aubergine! I said no, then I found myself looking at a bag of popcorn for £1.25 which seemed reasonable. I went back and got the aubergine.

I've stocked my freezer with vegetables for years, because migraine meant I often had to throw out fresh fruit and veg, and now I've also added frozen mango and frozen chestnuts so I can make scrummy healthy things.

Don't cut back on healthy fats, like olive oil, and particularly coconut oil which may also reduce insulin resistance.

With proteins, like beans and nuts, my rule of thumb is to go nuts for nuts, as they are full of healthy fat and protein, and are low GI, but for beans, which are also great, I try to stick to eating them more at lunchtime as I find digesting them at night can cause more hot flushes.

Don't fall for "healthy" and "natural" labels – really look hard at what you are buying and eating. Most of the time, when I eat poorly it's because I'm tired, rushed, haven't planned properly or I'm hungry. Now I always carry a bag of nuts which helps, but having healthy homemade dinners and snacks in the fridge and freezer makes healthy eating really easy.

My body is changing and yours will too, so keep refreshing what you know about what and how you eat. I'm hesitant about eating less, because blood sugar lows were a common migraine trigger, but I'm going to start experimenting with eating lighter in the evenings and see how it makes me feel.

It's all about learning to eat like an athlete, because we are all athletes.

11.   Consider turning down the thermostat

After my research on hot flushes and brown fat (or brown adipose tissue) …and beige fat… it seems a good idea to try out the idea that as little as 2 hours at less than 19 degrees can help activate our brown and beige fat, perhaps use calories to generate heat and increase insulin sensitivity.

There's also the possibility that this could help convert more white fat to beige, stop our brown fat turning white and prevent type 2 diabetes.

I don't know about you, but 19 degrees is quite warm for me (unless I'm ill) and the NHS recommends heating your home to only around 18 degrees even if you have health issues or are elderly.

**12.	Every day is a new day.**

Keep going and keep improving, learning from what you are doing.

Everyone is different and your results will no doubt be different to mine – they're different to what I expected.

a.	I didn't expect it to be so painful – sorry but that's the truth!

b.	I didn't expect it to prevent and minimise my migraines so fast. If I had, I would have done this years ago.

c.	I didn't expect the huge jump in my energy levels after a week or so – that was a pleasant surprise!

d.	I didn't expect not to lose *any* weight at first. That's still very slow going. I guess I'm coming from a lower place than I've been in a long time, but I can start to see my trousers falling down – my hips are a lot more toned, as are my arms, so I'm guessing the belly weight loss is on its way. Don't jump on the scales too soon, once a week or once a month will probably be more encouraging.

e.	I didn't expect to fall in love with healthy eating the way I have. Once I made the connection between insulin resistance and migraine, "treats" stopped feeling like treats, but the ability, the energy and lack of migraine to plan and cook healthy vegan meals is just mind blowing for me. I have homemade vegan risotto with cashew cream and chestnuts in the freezer, I have homemade vegan korma with coconut cream in the fridge and freezer. I've made spring green crisps! I make mango and spinach smoothies. I feel like a new woman. And I'm loving it.

13.   Enjoy life.

I've had to give up coffee and alcohol because of migraine and perimenopause. I'm looking forward to the day when I can enjoy a glass of wine or a cappuccino (almond perhaps). I look forward to going out and seeing my friends, being able to travel, even just up to London. I look forward to being able to eat spicy food and not have awful hot flushes. I look forward to being able to put on those jean shorts that I bought a few years ago (I know they were loose back then.) I look forward to not having to make excuses or cancel plans because I have yet another migraine. I look forward to looking in the mirror and seeing me, happy and healthy staring back, but in the meantime, I look in the mirror (or if we were in the same room, I'd be looking at you) and who I see, what I see, looking back at me is a warrior, and I couldn't be prouder.

Everyone has their vitamin Z for Zumba (or should that be vitamin X for exercise?) It's that thing you love, that works, that is usually the last thing you try because you've tried everything else. For me it's dancing or Zumba. I love swimming and walking but my body sometimes needs the high intensity of dancing to stay healthy.

After giving my brother a kidney, it was belly dancing that helped me get my muscles working properly again and as all the kinds of dancing I love – salsa, belly dancing, African… can be part of Zumba, it works for me… most of the time.

I trained as an Instructor in 2010 and at one time was teaching 16 classes a week, including seated classes for people with disabilities, but I haven't taught full time since I left London in November 2016.

November 2019. I've found a place to rent back in England – finally! I make the arrangements while I'm in Rome visiting my friend, hands shaking because I haven't lived in one place for more than a few months since November 2016. It's been a long road. While I'm in Rome, walking around a lot, I realise that I need more – I'm not that fit. When I get back to England, I'm going to start doing my Zumba DVDs. (As an Instructor I get a complete Zumba workout sent to me every two months, and I have about three years worth available online.)

When I get back to London, I do a workout for a couple of

days in row in the youth hostel where I'm staying. I also order some new workout shoes and gear in the Black Friday sale.

Finally, I'm on the South Coast in my new home, which is lovely and my landlord and landlady are great. It's only a winter let, but it will be a great place to get healthy and figure out my next move.

I come down with a terrible cough and cold. I go to the chemist and she gives me some cough syrup and tells me not to take any of the Lemsip as this year's cough is a dry one. Drink lots of fluids. It knocks me for six (but, not once, do I think it's Covid). For about three weeks I do a few things in the morning and then land on the couch for the rest of the day as I can barely move in the afternoon. I cough all night and struggle to make it downstairs to the bathroom. So much for Zumba. That's back on the back burner.

I hope I don't miss Christmas.

December 2019. My Zumba gear is in a big box under my Christmas tree. My landlady surprised me with a small, real tree and it's so cute. I've finally got my decorations on an actual tree for the first time since 2015. I'm in love with it all.

I'm well enough to spend Christmas Day with my family, but suddenly yank my shoulder and I'm in agony for the afternoon, evening and the next few days. The pain is so bad I can barely think about doing my physio exercises for my back, which I normally do every morning, let alone think about Zumba.

January 2020. Okay, let's try this Zumba thing again. If I do it every other day, I should get my fitness back up and maybe I can think about starting teaching classes again.

March 2020. So much. We get permission from Zumba Home Office to do classes online, so I email my previous participants (so glad I kept my mailing list going) and set up a few class times each week (I mean it's not like I'm going anywhere else!) My landlady gives me permission without hesitation. I'm glad I'm in such a lovely place. She's also given me a proper let and I've applied for Universal Credit as all my other work has disappeared.

I start classes at about the same time as lockdown and the same time I come down with Covid again. Luckily, even though I have to go to bed after each class, the movement keeps me going and perhaps it's the exercise that gets me through this week. My old class participants from different classes are meeting each other for the first time online, and we adopt one of my ladies' mantras, "Shit or Bust." I write it on a piece of paper and leave it in the kitchen for when I come down and am in despair.

I also spend a lot of time in the kitchen thinking, "What can I eat?" I've gone from no biscuits to six biscuits with a cup of tea before I can get out of bed. I'm not worried, this lockdown is only for a few weeks.

Summer 2020. Zumba Home Office have put on an online Zumba Convention! I'm going to do as many sessions as I can and give myself a boost.

I put my back out on like the second session. I'm gutted. I'm also really busy anyway, have been since the start of Covid as my family need someone who's not shielding to go the supermarket, get prescriptions and generally do anything they can't. My landlady and I remark to each other, when we fly past each other, how so many people say that they are bored since lockdown started – we're busier than ever.

I manage to watch some of the sessions anyway and catch the end of one on twerking one day, when I am feeling really down. The presenter cracks me up, it's just what I need, and I love that the first question in the Q&A is, 'How do I adapt this for my Zumba Gold class (the over 50s and people with health problems)?' Let's twerk! (As soon as my back recovers.)

Autumn 2020. My classes have become just one weekly Zumba Gold class with a small group of ladies. We're about five when we're all there. It's not a lot compared to when I used to teach 100-200 people a week, but it's our Monday morning get together, when we keep each other going and encourage each other. So much going on, and sometimes it's hard to navigate, to talk about what's going on without letting it descend into a moan and groan session. But really all I have to do is to get the music going and we cheer up.

The songs tend to be about getting together and seeing each other again, but there are some I can't do because I know I'll burst into tears. But we keep going and whenever I have Covid like symptoms I think it helps.

I've had to shield seriously so many times as a carer, accompanying my brother into hospital for essential treatment, it's become second nature, I'm such a hermit these days but I love my Zumba mornings because I don't have to think about 2 metre rules or not touching anyone, it's the contradiction of feeling closer to these guys every Monday than I do when I'm actually physically in person with anyone, being careful not to get too close. I'm exhausted.

December 2020. Some of my friends and at least one of my ladies spent Christmas alone. I was able to bubble with my mum and brother but was alone for Christmas Eve and Boxing Day. It's miserable but it helps me that I can get on the phone and be someone they can talk to. Misery loves company.

January 2021. I think I have Covid again. I get my first test in a major test centre (I've had all the others at the hospital in preparation for my brother's procedures). Thankfully I'm clear but I might be having a breakdown. I'm hot and sweaty, nauseous, I'm getting serious migraines beyond anything I've had for years. I'm struggling to get out of bed. I've been using meditation and everything I've learned to keep me going but I stand in the bathroom so many days not sure I can keep going. I've been going out for walks to the beach and hugging the trees, but my energy levels just keep dying, out of nowhere and now that we're not allowed to sit on benches, I'm scared that I might get hassled by the police or worse if I have to sit down. I'm scared to go for a walk. The only thing keeping me going is my Monday morning Zumba Gold class. I think it does more for me than it does for my participants – thank God they're keeping me going.

Summer 2021. It finally dawns on me that what I am experiencing is perimenopause. It's probably the nausea that makes the penny drop. I feel nauseous so much of the time and the only thing that helps is tortilla chips, ginger ale and sparkling water. My migraines have also changed, they seem to be a lot more frequent but not as painful – I'll take that, but sometimes the pain and nausea comes at the same time, especially first thing in the morning and it's really hard to handle. I try to go out for walks into nature like I used to do when I had really bad anxiety before I went travelling, but it's hit and miss.

Luckily, I registered with a GP before Covid, so I call them and manage to speak to someone one day when the nausea and pain is just too much. I've already been to the chemist and bought a pack of Migraleve, which I've managed not to take for over four years. It's paracetamol, codeine and an anti-nausea medication. Pain killers can give you rebound migraines but, as the GP says to me, 'You have to get through.' It's good to have the reassurance that I'm doing the right thing. She's also going to refer me for some tests to see if I'm actually menopausal and some tests to make sure there's nothing wrong with my uterus because my periods are so heavy and painful.

I've also put on a lot of weight because I'm struggling to have the energy to walk around the block so many days, but that seems to be the same for so many people.

January 2022. I get food poisoning. I am so ill I can't keep anything down, even water, for two days. I take to sipping three sips of water after I've been ill – anything more seems to trigger another bout of nausea. I feel awful and headachey and am so relieved when I can sip a second lot of three sips of water without being ill.

February 2022. I'm staying over to look after my grandma, but I get so sick I have to go home. I'm supposed to be taking my brother to hospital the next day, but I tell them they need to find someone else. 'There is no one else,' I'm told.

'There has to be, because I can't do it if I'm throwing up.'

True to form, I'm still throwing up again the next day, but in a way it's a relief to just sink back into bed, to stop trying so hard. I sip three sips of water like last time. It's bad, but this time I know what I'm dealing with.

Spring 2022. Finally, it dawns on me that I don't have a

recurrent stomach bug. It's migraines. I'm so used to having one kind of migraine, the really painful kind that only make me throw up because the pain is so bad, and then the second I had last year, where the nausea and pain come together, that I didn't recognise these, where the nausea and exhaustion is more like food poisoning. I was also thrown because I never used to get migraines when I had my period, just when I ovulated, but these bouts of nausea are closer to when I start my period. Every time I feel like I understand my body, it changes.

I've had to cancel so many classes and my family have had to cover for me as a carer. I feel like I'm apologising all the time. Sometimes I am over the migraine, but as I haven't been able to keep anything down for two days, there is no way I can teach a class.

I develop routines and coping mechanisms. I eat a lot of chips, they're often the only thing I can keep down. Sweet and salt popcorn helps too.

I try to walk for an hour each day, but on migraine days I'm lucky if I can make it to the bathroom.

My GP prescribes me an anti-nausea medication I can tuck into my gum when I can't swallow tablets and it seems to help and I can drink a cup of tea and sometimes even eat food. It makes those two day bouts of nausea easier to cope with and easier to rebound from.

May 2022. I can't have HRT yet apparently, so I chat with

my local chemist (they know me pretty well by now as I live around the corner and am always popping in to buy up their stock of face masks – sometimes they even give away the out of date ones for free). The lady in the chemist recommends Menopace and, after I check it out, I give it a go. I'm like a blooming rotisserie chicken at night at the moment. At times I think, "So this is how they came up with the idea of what hell is." The hot flushes dehydrate me, which triggers more hot flushes, migraines and, when the two day bouts of nausea hit, I'm in danger of drying out completely. I'm not looking forward to summer.

Summer 2022. I start to do more research on migraine. I've given up over the years because there's so little that helps. I managed four years without pain medication and that helped, I think they got lower, but with Covid and all the stress, plus the perimenopause, it's not surprising they've got worse. I discover The Migraine Trust.

It turns out that all the research about migraines has changed but some of it I should have known. Codeine is a bad idea. I take my last Migraleve tablet in June and swear off codeine (and then I buy one pack of cheap tablets, just in case it gets too bad).

I miss two of my best friends' 50th birthdays because I'm too sick. I cry a lot. I'm missing so much, on top of missing so much because of Covid, everyone else is getting back, getting on with their lives but I am not even coping. I need to find somewhere cheaper to live because I can't work a lot of days (or look for work) but I can't move while I'm in this state.

I've put on so much weight, but I don't even think about it, I eat what I can, when I can, when I'm not throwing up.

One month, I have a period that is so heavy and two days of such awful sickness that I look in the mirror and I am paler than I have ever been, my lips are blue. Looking back, I should have called a doctor, but I just carried on, and the next day I call the GP to ask for more help. She's not much help when I finally speak to her, she says, 'Well, when you finish the menopause, your migraines will stop too.' It's such an idiotic thing to say that I can't talk to her anymore and I give up on GPs (again).

In the heatwaves I survive, to be honest it's easier when everyone is moaning about being too hot, when the sensible thing is just to sit in the dark and work, when it doesn't seem strange to worry about being dehydrated and spray yourself with water at night. It's kind of like everyone is getting a taste of what it's like to be me – hiding from the sun and trying to sleep at night.

I start to chart my migraines and figure out what helps. I quit coffee and then tea. I have withdrawal headaches but then my pain and nausea go down a bit.

September 2022. Things all seem to come at once. I finally get the tests done that my GP was trying to organise last year. I'm okay, heavy and painful periods are just normal for me. I'm not surprised, but I am relieved.

The Queen dies and I head up to London to attend a migraine symposium run by The Migraine Trust. My first time in London since Covid, I walk around Buckingham Palace and see all the mourners lining up to pay their respects.

I've already started taking B2 and, although they reckon it takes three weeks to kick in, my symptoms immediately seem to drop dramatically (apart from right after my flu jab).

It's such a relief, to hear the top doctors talk about it, and I realise how many other symptoms I have that I never realised were migraine… or could be perimenopause, or could be migraine one day and perimenopause another.

It's also a relief to hear a lecture on the clinical pathway. I'm doing the right thing, starting with B2 and then magnesium if I have to, avoiding codeine and pain medication in general. So many times, I felt like I was at the end of my tether, but now I see I am just at the beginning of this journey, there's a lot more I can try.

They tell me about a lecture on YouTube about hormones and migraine and, after watching it, I figure out that it might be prostaglandins triggering my migraines so, as soon as I feel a migraine or period pain coming on, I take ibuprofen or eat stem ginger cookies and I finally stop throwing up for two days solid each month, which is just as well as "each month" now seems to be every 15 days. I've figured it out just in time for my periods to get increasingly erratic. But I feel more human.

December 2022. By some miracle, I manage to move house! I move down to my dream location, 15 minutes walk from the beach and I feel like I am convalescing from the last few years, recovering from Covid, Covid vaccinations (both of which, it turns out, make periods and migraine worse). On the day I move, I get my period, and then nothing for several months. I'm too busy with the move to chart my migraines, although they've not stopped, they're like the old ones, and I don't throw up anymore!

February 2023. Migraines are still a problem so I decide to start magnesium – it's 400mg, but I'm going to try to do it through diet, so make a list and look up what I'm eating and try to hit 400mg a day. (If that doesn't work, I'll go up to 600mg.)

March 2023. I get a five week cold and, when it hits, I get a hum dinger of a migraine (puking ensues which makes the tonsilitis I feel coming on much worse). It's not until April that I'll be able to take a walk without having to go to bed afterwards. Classes continue every Monday, when I can.

I'm gutted when my periods start again.

June 2023. And then they're back. After the reprieve, a "monthly" cycle of 10-19 days means that I am chronic, experiencing migraine just as many days as I don't.

The vomiting is back too. Thankfully usually only for one

day, and sometimes the medicine works, but it feels all too cruel that I am back to this cycle of getting knocked down and then trying to get back up each few days.

I go up to trying to have 600mg of magnesium a day and get some low dose supplements to help me out.

After one migraine which lasts 6-7 days, I call The Migraine Trust helpline and have a little cry on their shoulder. They suggest evening primrose oil and to switch my GP.

I'm struggling but feeling better that this year, when it gets too hot, I can walk down to the sea in the evening and have a swim. It makes life worth living. I also find that when it feels like I might have a migraine coming on, a swim in the sea seems to head it off. Maybe there is something to cold water swimming after all – although this is pretty warm water swimming.

I keep trying to lose weight but then a migraine hits me and sometimes I can't get out of bed for three days, then there are two days of shuffling up the road trying to make it to the beach.

Somehow, most Mondays, I teach Zumba Gold, but every time, I can't believe I make it through the whole class. I think it must be adrenaline and muscle memory. Once upon a time, my friend Anthony said that one class a week was maintenance, so I hope by doing one class a week and walking when I can, and the odd swim in the sea, that I can get through this vile perimenopause. As me and my sister remind each other, our goal is simply to make it through menopause.

August 2023. I have two really heavy periods in August and so many days of migraine that I'm not sure how much longer I can go on like this.

September 2023. I've changed my GP practice and finally get to see a GP at the beginning of September. Before seeing him, I revise everything I've learned about migraine so far. I watch Professor Anne McGregor's lecture on hormones and migraine and discover that I suffer from menstrual migraine with aura, but in perimenopause this means that I don't just have a migraine when I ovulate, but also when I have my period and that these migraines are longer, more severe and take longer to recover from.

It looks like the next step for me would be starting on something like Candesarten, which is a blood pressure medication, but it's been found to be helpful for preventing migraine.

He's very nice, but can't prescribe Candesarten, which I thought would be the best migraine preventative for me, but sends me a text with some other options and also gives me a repeat prescription for the anti-nausea drugs (which don't seem to be working very well, I seem to keep throwing up).

I'm also clinically obese, which he's not too worried about, and my blood pressure is a little high, but not bad.

I look up the drugs, one has a tendency to cause depression, which I could do without, the other depression and weight gain, which is not a great idea, but the other is an anti-sickness medication which looks like it might help.

Perhaps the migraines and periods will ease off as we come out of the hot weather.

I also do a bit more research on ginger and figure a stem ginger cookie is about the same dose they used in a study in the States where they found it had the same effectiveness as a dose of sumatriptan – a popular migraine pain treatment. Worth a go, so I pick up a few boxes of cookies.

It seems ironic that I'm now writing a book about health, but I keep reminding myself, you wouldn't want someone writing about something they don't have experience of!

Sunday 1st October. I can't say it's getting any easier, but something strikes me as I'm riding home on the bus. I don't have the bone crushing fatigue that I was suffering from last year. Okay there are still days when I can't get out of bed because of the migraines, and the hot flushes are back with a vengeance, but it's possible that I could do a little more exercise. And, after being annoyed at the suggestion that doing a little more exercise might help perimenopausal symptoms or migraines, it might actually be a possibility now.

After dinner, I go out and walk up and down the road until I can't walk any more. Maybe it'll be 5 more minutes a day, or 10, but it all helps.

I read an article on The Migraine Trust about exercise – it's so helpful and they understand that sometimes we don't want to exercise because we're scared of triggering migraines, but it can help. Time to give it a go.

Tuesday 3rd October. I have an eye test, and my prescription has shifted so much that my optician refers me for an urgent blood sugar test, a HbA1C to see if I'm diabetic or something. That's a shock. They won't even make up my glasses or book a contact lens check until my doctor does the test. I am just over the legal limit (in a good way) for driving, but it's been only a year since I had my contact lenses checked, so it's a shock. I book a blood test for the 11th and try not to panic.

Wednesday 4th October. I do an extra Zumba session. Hopefully this will get my weight down and help with whatever blood sugar issue I'm having. (Please let me not be diabetic already.) Classes: 1, classes in the last 7 days: 2, week 1.

Friday 6th October. A migraine hits – the nausea and pain is familiar, but it's actually not that bad – perhaps all the stuff I've been doing is working, maybe those 5-10 minutes of exercise are shifting things for me?! I manage to still do a walk to the beach, which I couldn't do most days with a migraine like this.

Saturday 7th October. I wake up in the early hours feeling awful. It's hard to distinguish if it's just hot flushes accompanied by headache and nausea or if it's a hormonal migraine. I eat a stem ginger cookie, take my B2, go back to sleep, try to eat a bit of toast, go back to sleep again, and then wake up violently ill.

I'm vomiting blood.

I call 999. I can't stop crying. I am properly panicking. They say they'll call me back. I call my sister who says that one of them can take me to hospital if necessary.

I practice breathing and wait for a call.

When the person calls me back for triage, they try to reassure me that the small amount of blood I've puked isn't exactly what they mean by "vomiting blood" but it doesn't help me really, because I know that I could vomit for two days straight, so even if this isn't serious right now, it could easily become so.

I throw up again. I see dried blood. I call my sister and ask them to take me to hospital.

I wonder if I am overreacting as I pack a bag and close up the flat. Then vomit again and see more dried blood before my other sister arrives to take me.

There is waiting at the hospital, and tears, and just a little bit more vomit in the next few hours. There is so much kindness, from people in the waiting room who see me looking pathetic and in pain, and from the triage nurse who tells me that I'm okay, checks my blood pressure and tells me that normally they'd send me to the urgent treatment centre, but I'd have to wait another four or five hours, so they'll see me in A&E. There is so much kindness from the doctor who finally sees me, who tells me that the blood is probably from the lining of my stomach or oesophagus bleeding because I've puked so hard, but it's nothing to worry about, there is no magic wand and he wishes he could do more for me, but he'll do some blood tests, give me some anti-sickness drugs, some fluids as I'm dehydrated and then some pain medication (nothing exciting, just paracetamol, ibuprofen and maybe some naproxen). They'll also run my HbA1C to check what's going on with my blood sugar (or maybe it's a different blood sugar test… I'm not sure).

Finally, they manage to get a cannula needle in my hand and inject me with an anti-sickness medication called metoclopramide. After all my research on drugs and side effects, coming in to A&E all I could think was, "Give me anything, I don't care." They hook me up to an IV of fluids and leave it to drip into me.

It's not long later that I decide I've had enough. The nausea has finally stopped and so, as I look at the fluids dripping into me, I know I could do it faster with herbal tea bags and a bit of toast and Marmite. I'm also starting to feel panicked by the surroundings and, although the noises have been painful since I arrived, now the lights are starting to get to me.

The doctor agrees that I can take my IV outside for some air, and a little while later, agrees, that as my blood tests are all okay and I'm not feeling sick anymore, I can go home – although I have to sign that I'm leaving Against Medical Advice. Finally, I get home, drink tea and lie down in the dark, quiet and sleep.

Monday 9th October. I fully intend to teach Zumba, but most of my ladies can't make it and the one who can isn't feeling great. We decide I'm better off focusing on calling the GP and trying to get myself sorted. I convince them to prescribe me the metoclopramide tablets and walk over to pick them up – it's just over an hour walk, but I have to get the bus back, I don't have it in me after this weekend.

Classes: 0, classes in the last 7 days: 1, week 2.

Wednesday 11th October. I get my official blood sugar test done at the doctors. I also check my weight. I'm 91.5 kg. If I can lose 14.9kg, I'll just be overweight and not clinically obese. There's a goal. I walk all day. To the doctors, around town, to the hospital for my brother's appointment and around town some more. I have blisters. Tomorrow, I'm doing Zumba.

Classes: 0, classes in the last 7 days: 0, week 2.

Thursday 12th October. I've decided to treat Zumba like a physio session. It may hurt, it may make me feel sick and tired, but if it's the only thing I can do in the day (aside from my actual physio exercises) perhaps it will be worth it.

It's going to take some time for my blood test results to come in and to be able to talk to a GP about them, to get my new glasses and contact lenses and to talk to a GP about my migraines (I'm thinking about asking them for a HRT solution just for the hormonal migraines) but today I can do Zumba. If I can do it, I will.

I do the whole session, a whole Zumba Instructor volume online. I feel exhausted afterwards, migrainey and nauseous. I'm shot for the rest of the day and lie on my bed, although I don't go to sleep. I take one of my new anti-nausea tablets and I don't throw up. This is how I feel a lot of Mondays, but I'm hoping if I push myself, if I treat this as rehab, I might get through this stage and actually get fit again. And not be diabetic.

Classes: 1, classes in the last 7 days: 1, week 2.

Friday 13th October. I was such a mess yesterday that I decide I need to do everything urgent before I start. I'm still feeling migrainey, which could have been the exercise, or it could be an ovulation migraine – it's about that time. I do a short walk to the beach and back to get some air, I didn't get out yesterday and then get ready for Zumba. My ankle was sore afterwards, as well as my back, this is normal, for injuries and weak spots to flare up, but I'll wear my Zumba shoes for a bit more support.

This time, the exercise gets rid of the migraine, but then it sort of comes back and I'm useless for the rest of the day, but I did everything important this morning. So I do some baking, standing up until I have to go lie down again.

It's a nice feeling, I can feel where my muscles are getting more solid again and last night I slept for 8 hours straight – with no hot flushes or night headaches, which was brilliant. Unfortunately, tonight the hot flushes are awful. Maybe they have nothing to do with how much exercise I'm doing, but if I can stop throwing up for at least a week, perhaps I can keep my Menopace down for a whole week and that might help them?

Classes: 1, classes in the last 7 days: 2, week 2.

Saturday 14th October. I feel raring to go this morning, but hold back on the Zumba to get out for a walk as it's a beautiful morning. I do a slightly longer beach walk but am tired when I get back. I do some work and then a Zumba session after a "lunch" of porridge, walnuts and banana, which I've been having every day after or before my workout. I also have a bag of crisps.

I'm a bit nervous as I feel a bit headachey, but it eases off quickly when I warm up and the only danger of throwing up is through exertion. Gosh it's been so long since I felt like that – it's kind of nice, if you know what I mean.

One thing I have noticed and keep reminding myself is that so many of even the official Zumba workouts don't really warm up properly. I've injured my shoulder before doing one of these, so I make sure to really go easy on my arms and shoulders in the warm up and make sure they're ready before I go for it – same with any running or jumping. I play it safe in the warm up because I really don't want any injuries, but it's amazing how much I can do during the work out safely – lots of heavy duty working out of my arms and shoulders – if I don't push it too soon.

The other thing is to remember to go evenly when I'm doing anything with my hips – it's too easy to just go one way (the easy way) and strain my lower back. In my choreography I make sure I make it big and go both ways, or I used to remind people in class when I saw them just favouring one side. I've seen people just stretch one side of their body at the end – and then repeat. We fool ourselves because we don't want to stretch the tight side or have to balance on the weak leg. 'Keep it honest,' is what I say.

I try to watch "Strictly Come Dancing" in the evening, but the movement of the dancers and cameras makes me headachey and nauseous, still a bit too much migraine activity going on. I'll watch it on catch up when I feel up to it. At least I'm not in A&E this evening.

Classes: 1, classes in the last 7 days: 3, week 2.

Monday 16th October. I gave myself a rest day yesterday and ran around the family. Dropped thank you apple crumble off to my sister (for taking me to the hospital) took my brother over to my other sister for a visit, went to see Grandma and made her lunch, back to hang out with brother and sister and then flying kiss on the cheek with mum before heading home again and cooking a very healthy bubble and squeak inspired traybake with loads of chickpeas (maybe too many chickpeas). Turns out they're packed with magnesium so good for avoiding migraines.

Yesterday my body still felt stiff. This exercise is tough. I am reminded, because I'm feeling a bit headachy and nauseous most of the time, that as soon as we start losing weight we can get detox headaches, because the fat loss releases toxins into the blood. Oh fun. Maybe I'll get a little hit of coffee from last year – that would be nice.

My back is stiff all the time, where I strained it after I gave my brother a kidney. It's in the healthy zone of working out weak areas, but I have to be careful not to slip that disc and so I do a lot of miracle bends (from Kundalini Yoga, just stretching back into it).

I think I have to look at it like stopping drinking coffee, and tea, and having a week of withdrawal headaches – it will be better in the long run. I hope.

I have my class this morning, I'm teaching, but if I feel up to it, I might add some more Zumba training at the moment. I've been doing 45 minute sessions, but maybe I can bump them up and kick through this detox period a bit faster. Onwards and upwards.

Doing my own class is so much tougher than the others – partly because I know all the steps, so I put in a lot of energy! I add four more Zumba Gold songs at the end (just for me) from the Zumba website – gives me a chance to try new things and keep my workout going – but that's enough. I find my back muscles are growing and are fighting with my back fat – feels like there's too much going on there when I try to stretch. I know I will put on weight before I lose it as the muscles build, but I feel really tight and heavy. Maybe I should add some swimming into my program?

I know it sounds like I'm whingeing (which I am) but it has been so hard having headaches every day and not knowing if I can risk even reading my emails, or if they'll escalate into a full blown migraine and the exercise seems to be making it worse, for now. It's hard and I have to remember why I'm doing this. Maybe it will make the migraines better, but I will definitely lose weight and hopefully push back diabetes (and get my blood pressure down). One of the good things I noticed yesterday is that I didn't really have to snack so much, exercise does help us regulate our blood sugar, so maybe it's working already and that will help me not to have migraines when my blood sugar gets low. Eating six small meals (or at least snacks) a day has been shown to help reduce migraines, but it can be hard to do that healthily.

I'm also grumpy because I have to vacuum and it's so hard to do that without triggering a migraine.

I'm hoping I can squeeze in a beach walk later.

I do! And sitting on the beach, I check my test results – theyre in! And I'm not diabetic! Not anywhere near, I'm slap bang in the middle of normal. Phew!

Which means… I can call up my optician, book a contact lens check and maybe get some new glasses. It's a red letter day!

Classes: 1, classes in the last 7 days: 4, week 3.

Tuesday 17th October. Migraine. It starts at around 1am and it's a stonker. I feel awful and my hot flushes are off the chart. The migraine pain and nausea comes with the hot flushes, so I'm not sure if it's a proper migraine or the mini ones I sometimes get all night. Around 3am, I feel really nauseous so take one of my new anti-nausea pills. Around 5am, I have a cup of redbush tea and a stem ginger cookie. I wake up around 6:30, almost time for another tablet. Man, the nausea is hideous. I take the next tablet at 6:55am, five minutes early. I manage another cookie a little bit later and my B2 tablets with a green tea. I sleep in between. I text my mum to say I'm not coming over to paint, then my landlord to say he can't come over to paint and then the optician (who I'd managed to book a last minute contact lens appointment with) to say I can't make it. This is why I usually only try to do one thing each day, then, if I have to cancel, it's much easier. I use one of my old anti-nausea tablets, the ones that go in my gum (the pharmacist said I could) and I try to sleep again.

I wake up about 1pm. 12 hours from when it started and I'm feeling okay. Maybe it's the drugs (and not throwing up) or the exercise, but I feel not too bad at all. I manage to eat some food and even get a load of washing out on the line and sit for a while in the garden. I think a shower is too much, but I do go for a walk, aiming for the end of the road and end up on the beach. I even eat a proper dinner. Hallelujah, something is working, but these migraines usually last for 3-7 days, so I'm going to wait and see how I am tomorrow before I get too excited.

Classes: 0, classes in the last 7 days: 4, week 3.

Wednesday 18th October. I'm still feeling okay. Always that little niggling of a migraine in one side or the other, but as low as it usually is. Hot flushes are still bad but nothing like the night before.

I tentatively get ready to do some Zumba. I even manage to do some work beforehand.

I do an old ZIN volume I've done before, which makes it harder because I do more of the moves, and then even manage another four Zumba Gold tracks (they're a bit slow, so they kind of work as an extended cool down).

Classes: 1, classes in the last 7 days: 5, week 3.

Thursday 19th October. I'm very excited as I've managed to book a contact lens check and sight test with Vision Express (free as I get my lenses with Lenstore) so I am making it my mission today to sort out my glasses. Here goes.

My prescription is completely different again! It's very close to the glasses I already have. At first, looking at the sight chart, wearing my contacts, I can't read very low, and the optician tells me I'm not legal to drive. I panic and blink a bit and then I can read, almost all the way down. She reckons that perhaps I'm not correcting for my astigmatism anymore and I need different lenses. It's all very stressful, although she's very nice. She tells me it's got to be an underlying health issue and I need to go back to the doctor and get them to run more tests.

I go back to the optician from before and tell my sorry tale to Paul, the dispensing optician, who reckons that the contact lens issue is probably dry eyes, and I need to use some eye drops. That makes sense. I have eye drops, I just don't like putting them in when I have my contacts in. (That and I've been running the dehumidifier to try to get rid of the condensation on the windows… maybe a bit too much.) He says he'll get the optician to call me.

She reaches me when I'm on the bus, I've given up for the day and I'm going home for a cry. She explains that what has happened was what she was worried would happen. I've had a spike in blood sugar which has temporarily made me more short sighted. (This would tally up with the doctor in A&E saying my blood sugar was high.) Although my HbA1c was normal, it's an average, so wouldn't necessarily register any spikes which could affect my vision. I really do need to have a chat with a GP. (Easier said than done.) I call the surgery and they recommend I try to book another non-urgent appointment, although I do have one booked for next Friday. At this rate, I'll be booking them pre-emptively (I'm sure that's what some people do.) Or I can try an online consultation at 8am, but they only do about 10 of them so I'd better be quick! (I was sure I did one before, but didn't realise you could only do them at 8am… I keep learning.)

So fed up, all I can do is Zumba! (Although I've strained one of my pectoral muscles by going for it yesterday, so this session is only gently sweaty.)

Classes: 1, classes in the last 7 days: 5, week 3.

Friday 20th October. I send an early online consultation request to my GP surgery, then get ready to do Zumba. I get a text back saying that what my optician told me is "medically impossible". Not from the NHS website and from a mathematical standpoint… oh and the blood test I had in A&E. Ho hum. I email my optician and ask for what to say to the GP. I have an appointment next week, so I'm just going to bumble along until then. As far as I understand it, I'm safe to drive and maybe things (as well as my eyesight) will become clearer in a few days.

I'm not a stranger to being told I'm just a hysterical woman by the GP… migraines, perimenopause, depression… oh, how many times I've been told to go away because I'm imagining it. And how many times they've made me have painful tests because my "normal" isn't within their "normal" parameters.

I've also just discovered on one of the web pages I've been surfing that it only takes three days of inactivity to reduce insulin sensitivity, which reduces our ability to manage blood sugar. So many times I've been incapacitated by a migraine for 3 days or more. Generally, my migraines last around 5 days, and I would never have done a Zumba session when I was experiencing symptoms.

I also discover that one of the treatments for hyperglycaemia is to exercise at least five times a week because exercise increases our sensitivity to insulin (even if we don't lose weight) so it's easier to manage our blood sugar.

I feel weird in the afternoon. I walk to the beach and one minute I feel I could go back and do another Zumba session, the next I feel tired, nauseous and headachey. Maybe I'm eating too healthy? On the other hand, I did a 45 minute session today, whereas Monday, Wednesday and Thursday it was an hour. I also felt rough last week doing 45 minutes (but I was struggling to do that). Maybe I'll aim for an hour from now on – see if that makes me feel better?

I also chat to my mum and we agree I'll call Renal on Monday. I'm under them as I'm a living kidney donor and blood sugar spikes can be damaging to the kidney (I only have the one left). If they tell me not to worry, I'll stop worrying.

It also strikes me that, although I'm frustrated with the GP and not knowing what's happening and the hell I've been going through with migraines, it's no one's fault. It's not the GPs' fault that

I suffer from migraines or hormonal issues. It's great to feel that I might be able to do something to help myself, but a lot of my emotions are just fear – fear that this hope is ill placed, that I'll be back where I was in a few days, or that it might get worse. As wonderful as the hope is, I've also been here before with B2 and green tea and Menopace and magnesium… I'm better than I was last year but I'm scared. Perhaps the most important thing I can do right now is meditate and deal with that fear.

Classes: 1, classes in the last 7 days: 5, week 3.

Saturday 21st October. Today I attempt a grand feat. One hour of Zumba and then up to visit Mum, my brother and Grandma… and then round the supermarket on my way home. I'm starting to feel like I do normally – knackered and worried that I'm about to have a migraine. I do get a headache, but only about a 3 out of 10 and make it home, where I cook a healthy dinner and crawl into bed. I am pushing the envelope and can't wait for a lazy Sunday.

Classes: 1, classes in the last 7 days: 5, week 3.

Sunday 22nd October. I find my Lazy Day surprisingly busy. Now that I have a little more energy, it's amazing how many little jobs I see around the house that have escaped my notice, or rather, been on my to do list (some since I moved in). I make it for a beach walk and then… after I've made and eaten a very garlicky bean dip… do an hour of Zumba. Shower, eat healthy (although too many chickpeas) and crawl into my bed.

Classes: 1, classes in the last 7 days: 6, week 3.

Monday 23rd October. Zumba Gold with the guys. I stick to 45 minutes this time. Later, I call the Renal department. We have a long chat, and they're happy that I'm okay and that I'm probably not having sugar spikes that would be damaging my kidney. It is a little odd, they agree, and we agree that the best thing I can do is what I am doing – everything I can to avoid being diabetic and having any more sugar spikes and have a chat with my GP about my eyesight and general health on Friday.

Classes: 1, classes in the last 7 days: 6, week 4.

Tuesday 24th October. It's not a rest day because I'm going over to do DIY at my mum's house – there might be a Zumba later.

There's not. I'm too tired to even shower.

Classes: 0, classes in the last 7 days: 6, week 4.

Wednesday 25th October. I do pretty much what I did last Saturday – Zumba, visit Grandma, go to Emsworth to source paint for Mum's house, then to Mum's to help out with the boiler service, my brother and some of his other needs. I get home around 6:30pm, but unlike last Saturday I don't hit the ceiling of my energy, I don't crawl into bed in pain. I'm okay. Wow, this is what it used to feel like to be me. Grandma says it as we're saying goodbye, 'It's good to see you looking better.'

Classes: 1, classes in the last 7 days: 6, week 4.

Thursday 26th October.

Classes: 1, classes in the last 7 days: 6, week 4.

Friday 27th October. Class. Doctor… who is exasperated as he shows me my HbA1c result, 'It's not just good… it's… perfect! You have absolutely no risk of diabetes.'

'But, but, but… what about the opticians, what about the A&E doctor, what about the blood sugar spikes?'

'Well,' he says, 'you will have blood sugar spikes – if you get stressed, your cortisol will change. I mean, if there were a lion in this room right now… whoof, you'd get a load of blood sugar.'

So although I still need to figure out my eyesight – the dry eye and maybe even get another eyesight test… I'm healthy and I will figure it out.

As for the migraines, I try to explain that I think I'm having hyperglycaemic migraines caused by drops in oestrogen causing sugar spikes (as well as those lack of sleep issues and stress) but he is less than convinced. Because, as for hypoglycaemia, the clinical term hyperglycaemia has some pretty high numbers attached to it. But I realise, as I'm explaining, that I'm not talking about the clinical level or definition. My level of insulin resistance might not be an issue to someone who doesn't suffer from migraines, just as sunlight, noise, smells might not be. But that slight drop or high, which in a normal person would just be enough to say, make them feel hungry, or even hangry, or… with a high, make them feel fatigued, nauseous etc. can trigger a migraine for me. (And maybe a lot of other people who don't realise it.)

On the one end, what I am saying is highly researched and scientific. On the other, I am talking about an area where no one has put two and two together yet. That lack of insulin sensitivity, way, way before it becomes a clinical problem, is enough to ruin some people's lives, like mine, to take away our quality of life.

And what I am doing is working, I'm getting my energy back, I'm putting my migraines back where they belong – a rare occurrence, not a daily battle, I'm getting back my muscles, my healthy appetite (not just eating whatever I can manage to chuck in the oven and keep down to hold off the nausea) I feel like I'm getting me back, and my sanity, my hopes and dreams.

I also feel like I've been hit by a bus a lot of the time as I'm getting a lot of DOMS (delayed onset muscle stiffness, or is it soreness) but I finally feel like I've found my way and I'd be an idiot to stop following it now. (I just have to remind myself of this when I feel like taking the time to do the Zumba is selfish and inconvenient!)

I also get on the scales, I've lost…. 0.2kg, maybe. (I do take my boots and jumper off, so it may just be the weight of the jumper!) But I expected this, as I'm building so much muscle. My real test is an old skirt, which I could just about get on at the beginning of this. I think it's a little bit looser, but each week I'll try it on and hopefully I'll start to lose that belly fat (it's becoming belly and back muscle!!)

I leave the doctor thanking him profusely because we've had a long appointment and a lot of laughs. He's newly qualified and I tell him I'm a good patient as I'm weird! I thank him for prescribing the anti-nausea meds and I'll come back to them if I need more. We talked about HRT, but it's not an option for me right now and here's hoping I won't need it!

Then I jump on the bus and the train and go do some serious DIY at my mum's house.

Classes: 1, classes in the last 7 days: 6, week 4.

Saturday 28th October. Classes: 1, classes in the last 7 days: 6, week 4.

Sunday 29th October. I think I've been having my menstrual migraine the last few days, but the pain and nausea only hit a 1 or 2, which I might not have even noticed if I wasn't bracing myself for it. All while running around and doing DIY at my mum's. I'm exhausted in the evenings and eat dinner in bed, but this would normally be 6 days out of my life. It's working.

Classes: 1, classes in the last 7 days: 6, week 4.

Monday 30th October. Classes: 1, classes in the last 7 days: 6, week 5.

Tuesday 31ˢᵗ October. I do feel a bit more migrainey than usual. It's tricky. Before, I would know when a migraine was coming on, these days, I so often have migraine activity that I have to risk it, even when I'm worried it might be a full blown one on the way.

Today I do a workout and then head over to do a bit of work at my mum's and then hopefully out with my brother and sister. It sort of works, but there are bus issues and train delays and the jobs turn out to be annoying and really hard work. In all the rush, I don't eat very well and for the first time in forever, I forget my water bottle.

But I'm feeling okay when I head home, trying to beat the weather coming in. We have storm warnings for the next few days. But by the time I finally get home on the bus, I'm all stressed out – like a lot of people, worrying about money. I emailed my original optician and they're happy that the second eyesight prescription (the one they didn't do) is correct, and so not that different from my current glasses and contacts. But I do want to get new glasses – my old ones are metal and are not comfortable to wear – especially when I have a migraine, so I've been eyeing up glasses in Specsavers. They tell me they have a 100 day guarantee, so I figure why not get a super cheap pair made up to see if they're any better than my old glasses? I can always get some more expensive ones later. Of course, the £29 ones I've been eyeing up aren't there, so while I'm waiting, I try on the £69 ones I was looking at before – at that price I could get free thinning or free transitions – so I could wear them instead of sunglasses. I can't help myself, they're just right! And then, of course, all the way home I stress out about the extra money.

Research on migraine has given us migraine sufferers one huge blessing – it's shown that often migraine is on the way long before we know it. So a lot of the behaviours, even foods we eat, aren't causing migraine, but are a precursor. So is my hour or so of stressing out and checking my finances over and over – instead of making the healthy dinner I had planned – a cause or an effect of the migraine?

I'm strung out by the time I get to bed. I've had some soup, done what I need to, but my head is hurting, I'm nauseous and I can't even watch TV. I take a metoclopramide tablet and am in bed by 9pm.

Classes: 1, classes in the last 7 days: 7, week 5.

Wednesday 1st November. Unfortunately, I can't escape this migraine by sleeping it off. I'm nauseous, so it might be menstrual, maybe the tail end of the one I've been feeling all weekend. Maybe I've been doing too much. Maybe it's the weather – I often get migraines when storms are on the way. I take another 2 metoclopramide tablets, 4 hours or more apart, and even a prochlorperazine, but I'm still a tiny bit sick. But really, nothing to write home about, after my usual migraine bouts of sickness. I sleep most of the day (probably helped by the tablets) but my stomach is a bit iffy and I am assaulted all night, all day… and then all night again by criminal hot flushes. Eventually, I decide to drink lots more water every time one hits (usually ever 1-2 hours at least) and by Thursday morning they seem to have died down a little.

Classes: 0, classes in the last 7 days: 6, week 5.

Thursday 2nd November. The wind blew hard all night, I look outside and there's a line of guttering flung halfway across the playing field. I hope it's not ours.

Everything seems to have worked, so I have a stem ginger biscuit and tea and can ignore the tablets. (Crazy how I forgot to try a stem ginger cookie Tuesday night – I would have if I hadn't been so stressed out. Time to slow down a little.) Normal, huge breakfast and by 9ish I'm working out. Not too hard, although still a Zumba workout I couldn't have done a few weeks ago. And then I add a couple more salsa tracks before I cool down, so it's a whole hour. The storm warnings are yellow today for wind and rain, so I'm definitely working from home!

Classes: 1, classes in the last 7 days: 6, week 5.

Friday 3rd November 2023. Finally, a break from the rain, like everyone else, I'm attacking the washing and getting out for a bit of shopping. I walk all the way along the beach, it feels like forever since I've been here. The shore is covered in seaweed washed up high by the storm. All the streams are full to the brim and there are new "ponds" in the field and the car park where the sea gulls swim – the waves are crashing on the shore, they're safer here.

I can't sit down because the benches are wet. I even have to shelter at one point under a tree, using my coat as a makeshift shelter for me and my rucksack. This feels more like my old life!

Finally, I make it to town and to Boots, where, I remember, there are a couple of seats. I'm knackered. I sit down and drink some water. The lady behind the counter comes out, 'Are you okay? Would you like some water?'

'No, I'm fine thanks, it was just a long walk, I needed a sit down.'

She comes back again in a few minutes, 'Are you sure you don't want some water – are you diabetic?'

'No.'

It's wonderful that I can tell her no, but it seems a strange thing to ask. I think I definitely need to keep on with this program!

I get the bus back, after my workout this morning and the walk, it's enough.

Classes: 1, classes in the last 7 days: 6, week 5.

Saturday 4th November. Another wet day, another weather warning. Today is a day for writing, reading and a really, really long workout!

I manage 75 minutes, which, considering I started at 45,

gasping for the end, is not too shabby.

Perhaps a bit too much, as I end up fighting a migraine later, before figuring out that I probably need a little more salt. Onwards and upwards. It's not great, but it's manageable with an early night. Not quite sure if I am pushing myself too hard – whether it's better to stick with a safer 45 minute workout or whether this is good – to get a long workout in the tank if this migraine was a hormonal one coming on anyway? Always the questions we ask ourselves about migraines – did I do too much and trigger it, or do too much because I could feel it coming instinctively?

Classes: 1, classes in the last 7 days: 6, week 5.

Sunday 5th November. Horrendous night of hot flushes, they're really getting me at the moment – roll on no longer being clinically obese and maybe I just need to hydrate better?

Oh, to black cohosh or not to black cohosh?

The hot flushes don't help the migraines, as my sleep is so disturbed, but come morning the migraine is all but gone and finally the sun is shining. I think it's a long walk along the beach (with shades of course) and a lazy Sunday as last weekend… well, I didn't really have a weekend as I've been catching up on so many things from the times when I had to cancel stuff from migraine. I catch myself this morning having forgotten important things, it's kind of nice, it's so long since I had a few days migraine free – when I have a migraine, I'm always checking my to do list, I'm so afraid of not being able to get things done.

"It's a new dawn, it's a new day, it's a new life for me,

And I'm feelin' good."

I try and have a bit more salt, but it's the lack of sleep that gets me when I get home, I can barely keep my eyes open. I try for a nap but that doesn't work, I'm still having the odd hot flush. I finally decide that I really can't manage Zumba today and eat and tidy everything up early so I can go to bed super early – 6:30pm – at least this way I can get some sleep, even if I have another night of terrible hot flushes.

Classes: 0, classes in the last 7 days: 5, week 5.

Monday 6th November 2023. I feel much better and not such a wreck when I stop sleeping around 5am (I'd say wake up, but I'm awake so many times through the night…) I'm going to try to keep turning the thermostat down, I'm basically cold and hot all night. I read the first study on hot flushes and brown adipose tissue – I think instinctively I'm on to the money with my speculation. But it annoys me, that they call hot flushes "bothersome", f*ing "bothersome"?! It's like torture.

I figure they were the worst on Saturday night, after I did a long workout. I think the exercise is building more BAT, supporting it, I think the hot flushes are probably something positive overall happening in my body, like the DOMS, but I think I also need to figure out how much I can take and still get through the day (and keep doing exercise). I need to find my balance. I figure as long as I am doing 45 minutes or more, five times or more in a week, that should be enough to keep increasing insulin sensitivity and developing BAT, without hopefully ruining my life with hot flushes.

And I think I need to try to hydrate – keep my salts up – just a little bit more. I think I need to make some more green crisps!

It's my birthday this week and I'm hoping to publish this book as well. I'm hoping to finally have a birthday that isn't locked down or marred by migraine, I'm keeping everything crossed.

I see from the memories on Facebook that it is seven years to the day that I left my home in London and went off on my Camino the day after my birthday.

When you walk the Camino, with a heavy rucksack on your back, you carry all the things you think you may need, water, warm clothes and a sleeping bag, food and medicine, until it feels at times that the weight of it will break you, putting it down for a time feels so wonderful, picking it up again feels impossible. Then you come to a place, where you find faith and the strength to be free, to let go of everything you don't need, you become an ultra-lite backpacker and you realise that all the things you were holding onto were just holding you back. You stop carrying your shoes and start wearing them, you stop carrying your water and just drink it, you stop carrying food that you no longer want just because you paid for it. You let go of the fear and embrace joy.

On this journey, you burn the energy already in your body, the fat your body carries in case you might need it. You find the exercise you love and you realise that far from seeking something distance, something outside you, the answer you were so desperate for, was within you all along.

Classes: 1, classes in the last 7 days: 5, week 6.

Tuesday 7th November 2023. OMG! So, yesterday, I couldn't stop worrying at the conundrum that is brown adipose tissue (and beige and that whitened brown stuff) and reading more and more scientific studies. This is the thing about being a mathematician, it's like an addiction, like being a detective, trying to figure out the logic, how it works… and I developed a theory – that actually it was the room being too cold that was triggering the hot flushes! I was so confident, that I turned up the heat in my bedroom, just for a few hours, before I went to sleep – and then turned it down to the regular temperature and guess what – I was toastie all night and only had a couple of small hot flushes – what a difference!

(I also had a really bad acid stomach from eating peanut butter on toast a bit late, I think I need to eat a bit earlier to make up for the hour time difference now the clocks have changed.)

In the night, even more becomes clear to me, my brain keeps working – I have another theory about hot flushes on top of my theory about why we have them in the first place. This is amazing and this could change everything!

I've got to publish this book – I can't wait to shout about this from the hilltops. Finally, a breakthrough in hot flushes!! After years of being fobbed off or being given choices that aren't really choices…

Best of all, it means I can exercise as I want to. When I wake up now, it's because I've actually had enough sleep! It's 6:42am and I've already had breakfast, so I should be able to work out by about 7:30am, which gives me ages to exercise and shower. I've got an appointment to pick up my new glasses at 10am – they're rose tinted! Before I go over to work at my mum's. (I'm going to surprise them with the glasses!)

I really feel like I'm getting my life back and, as much as I love sharing how to handle fear of success (and I'm gonna!) the experience of writing this book has been extraordinary. We say in the shamanic world that, as much as we read and study and learn from other gurus, the real truth comes from direct revelation. You'll see it in my other books, it's that moment I'm sitting on the beach at sunrise and truth arrives, and really it was something right in front of me, I just couldn't grasp it. Honestly, if I look at what I've written, all the studies done, and I add it all up and figure it out, it's the same thing – the combination of investigative reporter and listening to my inner wisdom that has brought me here and, you know, maybe what I am really doing is uncovering our fear of success as human beings, or at least one of them.

If the studies show that HIIT exercise is the best thing to

prevent type 2 diabetes, why are we not all doing it?

If healthy eating is the answer to so many illnesses, why aren't we doing it?

If health is success, why aren't we doing everything to be healthy?

In my case, I had created a very small window of what I thought was healthy, what I thought I could manage. And I'm so glad I've blown that window apart, and now, once again, the world is my oyster.

It's five weeks since that optician's appointment. I remember from the day I left my house in London to the day I reached Finisterre beach – the ending of my Camino de Santiago, it was 28 days, what they say it takes to learn a new habit, to embed a new lifestyle. I think, as well as getting started with the exercise, I needed to understand this about the hot flushes, because it was starting to get in the way, but I think, tomorrow it will be 28 days since I committed to *my* health and, although this journey is just beginning, I know I can do it.

Classes: 1, classes in the last 7 days: 5, week 6.

About the Author

Since 2010, I've been the Explorer-in-Chief of Pearl Escapes, the organisation I set up to share all the most wonderful things (escapes) I could find around the world. I've shared Zumba, traditional healing, spiritual practices, my own deeply personal story of being a kidney donor and my adventures around the world.

After studying in person with don Miguel Ruiz and his sons in 2016, I was fortunate enough to be able to complete an online apprenticeship with them during the pandemic.

I've studied with Beto Perez, the founder of Zumba® Fitness and the top Zumba Instructors in the world. My biggest achievement was rolling out Zumba Gold. When I began, there were no classes in my area of London, let alone chair classes – by the time I left there were 22 taught by other instructors.

I studied Maths at university because I loved the black and white of it, but then it started to become more complicated, less absolute and I couldn't handle those shades of grey, the spaces in the knowing. I got my degree but then walked away, falling in love with film, eventually getting a Masters degree and making a dance movie. Through Buddhism I learned to love the spaces in between, the mystery of life and this last practical experiment, this recent journey has shown me, magically that so many things come back around to the beginning, whether it's Maths (which is also problem solving) or the title of my feature film, because I've learned so powerfully, from the last few years, that we have "Everything To Dance For".

Acknowledgements

In this book, and in life, there are times when I can be awfully negative about modern healthcare, GPs and other health professionals. But I owe them my life and the lives of most, if not all, of my family, so I want to express my deep respect (underneath the glib comments) for the people who try so hard to keep us healthy.

It is a complicated thing we are trying to do, whether we are doctors or fitness instructors, we are following what we've learned and the previous research, at the same time knowing that there is so much more we need to learn.

I want to particularly thank the people who work so hard to help develop understanding of migraine – whether that is the neurologists or the people who work for charities like The Migraine Trust. Last year, when I had exhausted the support from my GP, which honestly wasn't much help, they were a lifeline.

I want to thank The Migraine Trust for giving me the confidence to start exercising seriously again (even though I was training every Monday) because they had an article online about how scary it can be to start again, when we are experiencing so much migraine activity and there is the danger that dehydration or low blood sugar could trigger another episode. I'm grateful for their very practical advice on how to start again. I really shouldn't have needed it after all of the experience I've had, but I did. I needed that gentle encouragement and support.

I'd also like to thank the GPs who put up with us when we

rail against the lack of research, the lack of support and understanding for migraine, menopause and all other kinds of health issues. I know that there are times when they would like to give us different advice or medication but have their hands tied by current guidelines.

And I'd like to thank the NHS in the UK for all the times they've been there for me. It is so hard to even consider prevention or helping people like me who seem to be healthy, but whose quality of life is so challenged, because so much of the resources are focused on keeping people alive – that's as it should be, but I hope, in some way, that I can do something with this book to not just shift the needle for my own health, but for all the people for whom insulin resistance is or is becoming an issue, and I hope that can help us all to stay healthier and need less medication and medical intervention to keep breathing.

Also by the Author

Books

Pearl Escapes Fear of Success series (self-help/business)

Pearl Escapes Fear of Success

Pearl Escapes Fear of Success Practical Trainings:

Pearl Escapes Fear of Success Awareness Training

Pearl Escapes Fear of Success Action Training – "Dip" Method

Pearl Escapes Fear of Success Analysis Training

Pearl Escapes Other People's Fear of Success Training

Pearl Escapes Fear of Success Action Training – "Dunk" Method

Pearl Escapes Fear of Success Development Training

Pearl Escapes Fear of Success Adaptation Training

How I Escaped My Fear of Success (workbook)

All Empires Fall (financial thriller)

Camino de la Luna series (self-help/travel) - available with photos as full colour paperbacks and colour pdf eBooks. The first few audiobooks are out now

Japan Is Very Wonderful

free Feeling Real Emotions Everyday

Camino de la Luna – Take What You Need

Camino de la Luna – Unconditional Love

Camino de la Luna – Forgiveness

Camino de la Luna – Compassion and Self Compassion

Camino de la Luna – Courage

Camino de la Luna – Truth

Camino de la Luna – Reconciliation

Pearl Escapes Guide to Healing & The Guide to Spa Breaks and Escapes from Pearl Escapes (various editions)

Meditation for Angry People

The Wee, The Wound And The Worries: My Experience Of Being A Kidney Donor

Pearl Escapes Mini-Guides (various locations)

Love And The Perfect Wave (romantic novel)

Please also check out my audiobooks, available on most platforms, particularly Apple

Movies

Everything To Dance For

More from Pearl Escapes

My websites: pearlhowie.com and http://pearlescapes.co.uk/

YouTube: Pearl Howie

Instagram @pearlescapes

Facebook: https://www.facebook.com/pearlescapes

https://www.facebook.com/pearl.howie1

Udemy: Pearl Howie

www.ingramcontent.com/pod-product-compliance
Lightning Source LLC
Chambersburg PA
CBHW050729260726
48661CB00001B/139